BUZZ

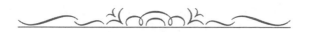

BUZZ

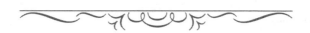

A YEAR OF
PAYING ATTENTION

Katherine Ellison

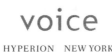

HYPERION   NEW YORK

Copyright © 2010 Ink, Inc. fso Katherine Ellison

Wechsler Intelligence Scale for Children, Fourth Edition (WISC-IV). Copyright © 2003 NCS Pearson, Inc. Reproduced with permission. All rights reserved.

"Wechsler Intelligence Scale for Children" and "WISC" are trademarks, in the U.S. and/or other countries, of Pearson Education, Inc. or its affiliates.

Library of Congress Cataloging-in-Publication Data

Ellison, Katherine.
  Buzz : a year of paying attention / Katherine Ellison.—1st ed.
    p. cm.
  ISBN: 978-1-4013-4088-9
  1. Attention-deficit hyperactivity disorder—Diagnosis—Humor. I. Title.
  RJ506.H9E45 2010
  618.92'8589—dc22

                                2009032677

Hyperion books are available for special promotions and premiums. For details contact the HarperCollins Special Markets Department in the New York office at 212-207-7528, fax 212-207-7222, or email spsales@harpercollins.com.

Book design by Karen Minster

FIRST EDITION

10 9 8 7 6 5 4 3 2 1

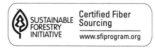

For Jack, as always,
and for my parents,
with love and appreciation

Contents

HOW ABOUT REFRAMABLE?

BUZZ

THE PREDICAMENT

"Understand Me!"

*For the moment,
what we attend to is reality.*

WILLIAM JAMES

A SEPTEMBER FOG HANGS OVER THE GOLDEN GATE BRIDGE AS I speed southward in our dented brown Prius. One son sits beside me, the other in the back.

Damn, damn, damn, I'm late again!

I swerve in time to avoid missing the exit to Highway 280, and gun the car toward Silicon Valley. The boys are out of school for yet another "staff development day," and I'm planning to drop them off with my parents while I have coffee with a friend and then meet with a venture capitalist who wants my help to write a speech. But I've left home so late I'll barely have time to give my folks a quick hello at the drop-off—sure to evoke their rolled eyes and weary headshakes.

Yikes! I nearly hit the car in front of me as my head turns to referee another potentially fratricidal fight. We argue a lot in my family. Except for Jack, my even-keeled spouse, we're moody, high-maintenance types. Which goes double for my eldest son, Buzz, who just turned twelve and each day fulfills my mother's old, cheerful curse. "One day," she'd say when I was growing up, "you'll have a child just like you."

A *noodge,* she meant, with a chronically urgent agenda, never able to take no for an answer.

My mother was right about that, and more. Three years ago, Buzz—the alias I've chosen for my son, for the electric-jolt way he usually affects me—was diagnosed with attention deficit/hyperactivity disorder (AD/HD), with a side order of oppositional defiant disorder (ODD). The first diagnosis signifies a problem of distraction and poor self-control. The second means that he is frequently a pain in the neck.

The point is, I have a certifiable problem child, while I'm also certifiably part of the problem. Call it diagnosis envy disorder, but Buzz's new status inspired me to check in with Dr. Y., the psychiatrist I first began seeing in my twenties, to ask if he thought I might share my son's disabling distraction. He said he did, indeed.

This alphabet-soupy new lens on our life helps explain our chronic chaos, but so far has done little to reduce it. Not that I haven't tried. Most recently, I've encouraged everyone in my family, including even-keeled Jack, to take fish oil supplements. Research suggests they're good for general brain health and mood.

Suddenly, Buzz squirms in his seat, tugs on the visor of his Dodgers cap, and announces: "I want coffee."

"Oh, Buzz," I say immediately. "You know that's not good for you."

"I NEED coffee."

He never drinks coffee. *Okay, I've let him have it maybe once or twice. But what was the final word on whether it stunts your growth?*

"Either coffee or a Coke," he growls.

Buzz is sitting up in front to minimize the risk of bodily harm to his nine-year-old brother, Max. Sometimes this works, but sometimes he gets upset and throws things or jerks back his seat to ram Max's knees. Will now be one of those times? My heart is expanding, and not in a good way. It seems to be pressing against my lungs.

"Neither one is good for you, and we can't stop now, as you know," I say automatically, switching lanes to overtake a slower car. My voice is wonderfully calm. *Hurray for me!* "We're on the *freeway,*" I add.

"COFFEE!" Buzz roars.

And, boom! My mind is off to the races. I should never, ever have given him Coke that first time—when was that again? To be sure, it's always there at kids' birthday parties; after age three, a parent basically loses control. But that's no excuse, since on several occasions I've bribed him with sodas for good behavior. And of course, I drink Diet Pepsi in front of him. . . . What a bad mom! But what if he needs it? I certainly need it. Could he be trying to muster his focus? Or is he just pushing my buttons—again? Oh, man, I'm never going to make it in time, no matter if we stop or not. Fantastic: late for the first meeting with a new client. I can't do anything right. And why on earth am I meeting my friend Pete today, when I should be using the time to squirrel myself away somewhere and finish the proposal for that book on plastic pollution that I promised my agent I'd deliver last month?

It is the autumn of a year in which America is involved in two wars, on the threshold of global economic crisis, and on course to a historic presidential election.

The radio news, before Buzz irritably switched it off, said the stock market is down three hundred points this week. *So much for the retirement fund! But why am I worrying about that, when bisphenol-whatever from plastic debris in the ocean is making its way up the food chain, and the Himalayan glaciers are retreating, threatening to leave several hundreds of millions of Asians without water? Not to mention the California snowpack—*

Buzz is still roaring: "I waaaaaaaaaant CAWFEE!"

I love Buzz and Max with a passion that continues to surprise me. They've helped make me a better person than I ever could have been without them. What I want most of all right now is to model healthy behavior for their sake.

"SHUT UP! SHUT UP! SHUT UP!" I yell.

"Mom," Max pipes up from the backseat, "I don't think the fish oil is working."

FEW THINGS IN LIFE are ever this plain, yet it's at this moment, following this latest train-of-thought wreck, that I take a breath, squeeze into the exit lane, and decide how I'll spend the next year. I won't write that book about plastic, after all. The topic is unquestionably important, but a project with a shorter deadline is vying for my limited attention. In this final year before Buzz hits his teens, I need to see if both of us can sharpen our focus and cool down our irritable ways.

That's how I get this wild idea. What if I could dedicate a whole year to just that goal? A year in which I'd put other work aside, making it my full-time job to seek the best path for a distracted parent intent on helping her distracted child. A year, in other words, of paying attention to attention.

I've always been good at deadlines. I spent more than two decades as a newspaper reporter and delivered my babies at ages thirty-eight and forty-one, timed with the last ticks of my biological clock. Now I look at Buzz, who, despite everything, occasionally still wants to be with me, and remind myself I've got at best another year in which he may yet want to learn what I have to teach.

And maybe there's something both of us can learn by looking through this attention deficit lens, murky prism that it is. Perhaps it can help explain my own history of unreasonable extremes: of screw-ups alternating with heady success, of buying high and selling low, and—so like my Buzz—of constant cravings for conflict and caffeine. It may even illuminate how I managed to win a Pulitzer Prize just three years after being sued for $11 million because of a careless reporting mistake, then realized my childhood dream of becoming a foreign correspondent, only to break my leg by running into a manhole in Managua while chasing Nicaragua's newly elected president—and did I mention that she was on crutches at the time?

Most urgently, I hope this new frame of reference can help me understand why I'm having such a tough time with Buzz. After spending most of my life feeling insecure about my smarts, I've finally, on the cusp of old age, come to trust them.

So why do I keep landing in these stupid situations?

· · ·

ATTENTION DEFICIT DISORDER, OR ADD—the popular name for a syndrome that has had at least five different names in as many decades—is a hallmark obsession of our frazzled era. It's simultaneously America's most commonly diagnosed juvenile mental disorder—affecting more than 4.5 million children, including nearly one in ten boys—and an increasingly trendy way of referring to aging adults caught between the rock of failing memory and the hard place of the modern data storm.

Nor is this phenomenon restricted to anxious Americans. Similar rates of clinical-grade distraction are being reported in other industrialized nations, including Japan and New Zealand. (Even China has become an important emerging market for Ritalin, although super-restless Chinese kids are still more often treated with traditional remedies such as acupuncture, herbs, and "dragon's bones," or ancient fossils.)

The field's leading experts describe the core problem as a weakness in the brain's inhibitory system: i.e., faulty brakes. Yet despite more than a century of dogged scientific research, the syndrome—diagnosed via a list of subjectively interpreted symptoms, including impulsiveness, forgetfulness, and distraction—remains elusive, with none of the straightforwardness of your garden-variety Down syndrome or schizophrenia. This fuzziness contributes to the fierce debate over whether many children are being needlessly labeled—which, most likely, they are, even as many other affected children surely aren't getting the help they need. What do we know for sure? Mainly that as each new label is bestowed, another set of overwhelmed parents must choose among a dizzying array of treatments.

Welcome to my world. It's a place swept by theories and therapies as contradictory as they are fervently held, running the gamut from medication to meditation; cognitive therapy to powdered soy shakes; neurofeedback, hair analysis, genetic testing, special diets, and summer camps dedicated to organizational skills. You can bet the house on costly, custom-designed exercise regimens to stimulate the cerebellum, tinted contact lenses, "eye movement desensitization and reprocessing," horseback therapy, swimming with dolphins, and, if all else fails, exorcisms. Your required reading list features such relentlessly optimistic titles as *The ADD Answer, Healing ADD,* and even *Dr. Bob's Guide to Stop ADHD in 18 Days*—all guaranteed to send an even minimally guilt-prone parent into riots of self-recrimination. Which promising new treatment have I still neglected to try? Or did I irrevocably blow it by drinking all that coffee while pregnant? Or by letting Buzz watch TV at age two? Did he eat too many processed foods; was I wrong not to have his adenoids removed; or did I hurt him most of all by sparing the rod? Is Buzz hopelessly spoiled, or an "Indigo Child," whose free spirit I should have more expertly nurtured?

And then there's the Drug Dilemma, which goes something like this: God forbid you medicate your distracted child, because you'll turn that child into a zombie, a midget, and/or a drug fiend, causing lasting damage to his brain that we'll only be able to measure once he's old enough to sue you. But God forbid you *don't,* because he'll fail at school, wind up friendless, lose all self-esteem, and/or self-medicate (i.e., become a drug fiend)—and blame you for your ill-informed parenting each day, after you drag home from work to find him, at the age of thirty-four, still lying on your living room couch.

Are we blessed or cursed by supposedly knowing so much more than our parents did? Especially when there's such fierce debate over nearly every aspect of what we think we know? Well-informed as we modern parents may be, we've ended up with much more data than knowledge, inclining us to burn countless megawatts of brainpower trying to discern that shifting line between character and disorder, explanation and excuse, "I can't" and "I won't."

MY HUSBAND, JACK, AND I have had as hard a time as anyone else in seeing our feisty son as disabled. There's no wheelchair, breathing tube, or special glasses. Instead, what often stands out at first sight of Buzz is his sparky charm: the soulful, long-lashed brown eyes, the quick mind, and the occasional zany joie de vivre.

Even his lapses of attention can be cute. There's that ready-fire-aim energy, that damn-the-torpedoes zeal. I remember him at age six, running the wrong way around the baseball diamond—much like me, as a daydreaming college student, crashing my bike into the back of a parked car. Our minds, apparently, were elsewhere, no doubt germinating seeds of creativity that might even flower one day. Still, despite that endearing side of clinical-grade distraction, and all the heady talk in recent years about it being a "gift," there's a great deal of evidence that it's anything but benign.

While many bright people have ADD, there's been no proven correlation with higher IQs. And for every proud poster boy, such as the JetBlue CEO David Neeleman, or the Democratic strategist James Carville, studies show that many thousands of others will wind up divorced, on drugs, and in jail. Sometimes it seems like there is no middle ground between glory and humiliation. Consider the case of swimmer Michael Phelps, who rose to international stardom at the 2008 Olympics, only to disgrace himself a few months later by being photographed with a bong.

Young adults with attention deficit disorder have four times as many car accidents as those who aren't affected. They have five times the rate of suicide attempts, and ten times as many teen pregnancies. They're also more than twice as likely to be arrested, and up to three times as likely to abuse alcohol and drugs. Add to this the huge financial toll on families and society, estimated at last count at nearly $30 billion in above-the-norm annual medical expenses. The disorder in children has been linked to significantly higher rates of divorce by their parents, and to a greater chance that the children will be physically abused. It may be invisible from the outside, but the suffering it causes is all too obvious.

BUZZ WAS AN EAGER, successful student right up until second grade: a typical time, as I'd later learn, for ADD symptoms to surface. It was then that he started forgetting to write down his assignments, or to do them, or to get them back to school. He lost permission slips, field trip forms, bulletins, thermoses, notebooks, sweaters, coats, and lunch boxes. Worst of all: he also lost every single member of his former pack of friends.

By sixth grade, Buzz was dressing the part of an outcast, with a daily uniform of Lakers basketball shorts and sleeveless shirt, touched off by a faux-gold necklace and oversized sunglasses. He chewed gum in class despite repeated detentions. His e-mail address was UpYours@hotmail.com.

At home, he turned his frustration on me, with an escalating series of relentless and impractical demands. He wanted his own bathroom, a trip to Fiji, a pet wallaby, and a Karelian bear dog—a breed known for its loyalty and hunting skill, which also sheds a lot, bites little children, and needs large spaces to roam. He refused to do chores or his homework, and wouldn't stop pinching and punching Max. Our conflicts escalated. Bribes failed; "consequences" backfired. Sent to his room, Buzz roared obscenities and threw shoes at the door.

At what I've come, I hope not too optimistically, to think of as our low point, Buzz, at age nine, went so far as to call 9-1-1 after I'd responded to yet another violent attack on Max by confiscating his Game Boy, the closest thing he had at that point to a stimulant medication. The police arrived within minutes, instructing Jack and me to wait outside the room while they investigated Buzz's claim of child abuse. My spouse and I stared at each other mutely—*Are we headed for jail?*—until I heard one cop's raised voice asking: "She took away your *what?*"

IT'S A MEAN TWIST OF FATE that clinical-grade distraction and its common companion—hotheadedness—are so often passed from parent to child, like flickering torches in a clumsy relay race. Family life can turn into a battle between the short- and shorter-fused, the provocateur and the easily provoked. I go back and forth from thinking I'm the best possible mother for Buzz, because I can so deeply empathize, to thinking I'm the worst, because we so often clash.

"Why do you have to argue so much?" I ask him.

"Why do *you*?" he'll retort.

I've downsized my foreign correspondent career, surrendering a penthouse apartment in Rio de Janeiro, to nest in the suburbs and be available for my children in the afternoon, while Jack, my newspaper-editor husband, works at his office in the city. I make snacks, drive to Hebrew school and swim practice, help out with the homework, cook dinner, and, ad infinitum, wipe off the toilet seat. But soon after the trouble surfaced with Buzz, crowding my days with conflicts and therapy sessions, my freelance work became both more necessary—to help pay for all those therapists, tutors, and lost clothes—and, frankly, a lot more alluring. Once the school day starts, I carry my steaming cup of coffee to the converted toolshed that serves as my backyard office, to work on magazine stories and consulting jobs. My shed, under an elm tree, is cool in the summer, cozy in the winter, packed with books and, in the mornings, blessedly quiet, always excepting those occasional urgent phone calls from the principal's office to come pick up my unruly child.

Work, when it's going well, makes me feel competent and in control, whereas with Buzz, no matter how hard I try, I seem to keep failing. Our conflicts eventually reach the point where my survival instinct is overriding my maternal instinct. I get headaches that only go away on business trips. I take more business trips.

I develop an expertise in environmental crises—climate change, pesticides, acidifying oceans—which, even while increasing my baseline anxiety, offer respites from the crises at home. Or at least they do until the day it hits me: I've come to love my firstborn child best of all when we aren't in the same room.

I mean, I adore him. I'd lay down my life for him. But it is just so hard to *be* with him.

Even worse, he seems to have figured that out.

With the stubbornness we seem to share, however, Buzz has kept showing me that my presence is needed, my worries aren't groundless, and more effort is required. As I write this, his troubles at school are continuing; the conflicts at home are unending; and my beloved child—who as a curly haired toddler used to dance through the market outside our apartment in Rio, sniffing the flowers in stalls where bemused vendors called him *beija-flor,* for "hummingbird"—recently left out a drawing for me to see. There was a rope, a noose, and poison, the drawing labeled, "Things I could use to kill myself."

How could I even begin to help him?

One day he told me.

On an afternoon about a year before the highway fight, Buzz was having a tantrum over something I refused to buy him. He called me an "asshole," ran to his room, and jumped on his bed, as I followed, yelling how he must never, ever use that language again.

Then, from under his quilt, I heard his muffled voice.

"Understand me!"

Understand him?

It seemed at first like another of his far-fetched ideas, the Karelian bear dog of mother-son relations. *My* parents never had to understand *me.*

Understand him? The funny thing is that by then, I already knew—despite all the well-meaning teachers, friends, and relatives who *already* thought I was spineless—that the best kind of parent for Buzz would be someone who could be just that calm and wise. And to be honest, I've always wanted to be more of that kind of person than the hothead I too often am.

Understand him!

How do I even start?

The Canadian psychologist Virginia Douglas, a pioneer in the field of attention, tells me that the duty of a parent of a clinically scatterbrained child amounts to nothing less than changing the flow of that child's life. On hearing this, I picture myself kneeling at the bank of a powerful river, shoveling dirt with my bare hands, and feel a mighty urge to go lie down and take a nap. But instead, I'm setting to work on the problem in the best way I know how. Within a couple months of the fight on the highway, I obtained a contract to deliver a book based on my dedicated effort, over the course of one year, to make our home more peaceful, help my son make the best of his particular brain, and maybe even Be the Change I Wish to See in Buzz. What follows is an account of that time—a year filled with ambitious plans, daring experiments, mood swings, random detours, more than a few blind spots, and occasional flashes of insight—in other words, a not uncommon sort of year for our shared neuropsychological profile. The key difference is that *this* year, I'm paying close attention.

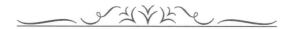

IT'S
PERSONAL

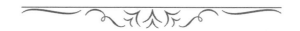

CHAPTER 1

HISTORY

Stuck on Input

Fall seven times, stand up eight.

Japanese proverb

WHOOSH.

Oh, no!

WHOOSH.

Ding!

WHOOSH.

Dammit!

WHOOSH. WHOOSH.

It's a cold October morning, midway through the first month of my year devoted to attention. I'm alone in a small, dark room, at a Buddhist retreat center high in the Colorado Rockies. A rubber cap studded with electrodes is stretched over my scalp to track my brain waves, as I take a "response inhibition" test to gauge my ability to pay sustained attention. My task is to mouse-click whenever I see a line a few pixels shorter than the line I saw when the test began.

WHOOSH is the sound the computer makes when I get it wrong—an airy strikeout pitch. The reward for getting it right is a melodic *Ding!*

But I'm not hearing many *Ding!*s. Mostly, I'm hearing WHOOSH.

This test was first developed during World War II to assess the vigilance of radar operators. It is so utterly beyond me that it feels as if an evil puppeteer has taken over my hands, while all the blood in my body is *whoosh*ing toward my head.

WHOOSH.

Ding!

WHOOSH.

Someone's screwing up here, but it can't be me. I'm too smart for that. Or so I've been told, whenever I've screwed up in the past.

Of course, this is just a simple neurological test. I'm not getting graded. The trick is not to get ruffled. Easy!

WHOOSH.

Shit!

"I'm done!"

Before I've consciously decided to quit, I've ripped off my cap and scurried back to the nice, light control room. I was supposed to stay in the dark room for half an hour, but I see by the clock that it has been less than five minutes.

Waiting for me in the control room is Cliff Saron, a tall, bearded neuroscientist based at the University of California at Davis. It was his idea that I take this stupid test. Saron is leading a major research project on the impact of meditation on attention, and I've traveled to meet him at this windy, remote refuge, ostensibly to write a magazine story, but really to find out more about whether meditation can help Buzz and me collect our scattered wits. After I confessed this to Saron, he suggested that his attention test would show if I were exaggerating my problem.

Well . . . nope.

"How'd she do, Tony?" he's asking Anthony Zanesco, his lab tech.

Tony is nice. Tony is my ally. Tony wonders if I need contact lenses, and did I have them in today? Tony observes that lots of people get frustrated with this particular test.

"She just walked out of there?" Saron asks, grinning.

I actually liked Saron when I first met him, a few months ago.

While interviewing him for another story, I ended up telling him about my troubles with Buzz. I don't usually complain about my kids with professional sources, but this was right after that 9-1-1/Game Boy incident, and I was still rattled.

"You just have to be calm," Saron had said. And somehow it registered then, in a way it hadn't before, what a big change that would be, just being calm. I wanted to know more.

Back in the control room, however, the goal seems farther away than ever. Saron is trying to get me to explain why I quit. Tony's right, he says, lots of people don't like the test. But they keep at it.

"I've only seen one person give up before you. She was one of my assistants. And she was terribly ADD. But everyone *else* manages to finish it. . . ."

Everyone else . . . I reach for my notebook, which feels familiar, though not in the cozy sense. Taking notes has been my main coping technique ever since I was a kid, fleeing my father's volcanic temper. On nights when he erupted, usually at some perceived disrespect from one of my two brothers, I'd grab my journal and run out the door to the garden of the vacant house across the street, where I'd sit at the edge of a concrete fountain and scribble the furious details of the latest melee until my heart stopped pounding. Years later, as I was reporting the news, my notebook again served as a shield raised between me and distressing realities: bloated bodies disinterred from secret graves in El Salvador; a runaway Amazon forest fire; the former Argentine terrorist-turned-businessman who coyly warned me not to write about him, saying, "Just as Hitler had his pet Jew, you can be my pet journalist." My notebook tells the world: "Hey, this is not *my* problem. This is *your* problem."

As I struggle to listen to Saron, however, the tactic is suddenly failing, and I'm scrawling messy half sentences. I've been joking about "my ADD" for more than a decade. I even joked my way through the appointment last year in which my longtime shrink, Dr. Y., diagnosed me. Yet until I botched this attention test, I somehow managed to avoid facing it this squarely: from having a funny excuse for losing my keys, it now looks as if I have a *brain disorder*. Were it not for the trouble with Buzz, I could easily have lived the rest of my life without applying this frightening phrase to myself.

So—just how grateful am I?

Saron is still talking, as I tune back in. "This is all about the world slowed down," he's saying extra-slowly, underlining his point. "You're pretty sped up. You're going to have to learn to be able to sit with your frustration, to see what happens on the other side of the pain."

As he goes on talking, however, my focus wanders off once more, responding to a chorus of new questions. *Whatever possessed me to think of spending an entire year focusing on this problem? Will all this attention to inattention end up making it worse? What harm might come from trying to weed the crazy garden of nearly five decades' worth of coping skills?* Soon Saron is completely drowned out by the WHOOSH of my craving to be anywhere but here.

THE BEST IMAGE I can think of to describe how it all too often feels inside my head is of a storm of Ping-Pong balls, each one suggesting a possibly better alternative to what I'm doing now. My father constantly told us: *Be in the right place at the right time.* But how can you ever really know the where and when of that? Even as I write this— weeks removed from that unsettling trip to Colorado, and back in my cozy garden shed, with a couple precious hours before the kids come back from school—I'm wondering if it really wouldn't be better to abandon this potentially embarrassing pursuit, sell the house, and drag the family to do something noble in Tanzania, assuming that's an option for two aging members of a dying media and two boys who still can't fix their own breakfasts. Or maybe I should write that book about plastic, after all. Or buy one of those new, flat-screen computer monitors. *Cliff Saron* has one.

Questions like these jam my synapses, even when I'm trying to listen to people I love. So how was work today, honey? *We still haven't hired anyone to fix the roof. It's been* two years, *and that weird stain on Max's ceiling might be mold. Mold!!! And we're running out of paper towels . . .*

And it's probably so much worse for Buzz. Racing through his preteen years with those weak brakes and none of the hard wisdom I've gained from all my own stupid crashes, he careens from impulse to action. Throw the tennis ball at his brother. Call me an "old hag." Eat seven of my calcium supplements at once, thinking they might help him grow taller.

There's that joke:

Q: How many kids with attention deficit disorder
    does it take to screw in a lightbulb?
A: Let's go ride bikes!

Speedy action equals relief—the only way to stop the option storm. It makes both of us do a lot of things we later regret—and helps explain why people like us have historically sparked such keen interest from doctors, philosophers, scientists, poets, and novelists. For millennia, these experts and artists have noticed us, diagnosed us, and occasionally treated us, yet never once cured us and rarely figured out how best to manage us. Instead—always barring those rare exceptions, when our out-of-the-box thinking has led to fame and fortune—society has blamed us, portraying our behavior as a physical defect, a moral failing, a family curse, or some ungainly combination of all three.

In ancient Greece, impulsive behavior was thought to be caused by an excess of red blood, with leeches, long before Ritalin, being the preferred treatment. In the Victorian Age, with its preoccupation with moral character, Charles Dickens drew an unsettlingly sympathetic portrait of a seriously distracted villain: the charming but terribly unfaithful James Steerforth, in *David Copperfield*, who ruins the lives of three women, most glaringly his own mother. It was in this same era that the psychologist William James presciently described the links between attention, distraction, and moral behavior, even as he doubted that much could be done to help people whose flickering minds led them to ethical lapses; while in Germany, a physician named Heinrich Hoffmann wrote a bit of verse destined to be cited in the literature of clinical distraction throughout

the subsequent century. It described a naughty boy called Fidgety
Phil, who:

> *won't sit still;*
> *He wriggles,*
> *And giggles,*
> *And then, I declare,*
> *Swings backwards and forwards,*
> *And tilts up his chair*
>
> . . . .
>
> *Till his chair falls over quite.*
> *Philip screams with all his might . . .*

. . . and you get the idea. In 1904, the poem appeared in the prestigious British medical journal *The Lancet,* coinciding with the dawn
of serious scientific interest in restless, disobedient children. By
then, the British pediatrician George Still had already embarked on
a groundbreaking series of lectures describing a group of his young
patients, who shared what he called a major "defect in moral control."
They were, as he said, distracted, overactive, accident-prone, aggressive, defiant, sometimes cruel and dishonest, and *strikingly insensitive
to punishment* (my italics). The bad behavior typically arose before
the age of eight and was more common in boys than in girls and, in
particular, in families that included alcoholics and criminals.

Still's research was pioneering in two ways. He defined, perhaps
for the first time, the cluster of annoying behaviors that today often
accompany a diagnosis of attention deficit disorder, and he also hinted
at a genetic explanation. The search was on for a smoking gun; in
ensuing decades, avid investigators would seek clues to the roots of
serious distraction with surveys, X-rays, brain scans, EEGs, and genetic testing. Today, if you type in "attention deficit" on PubMed, the
leading Internet archive of medical journals and reports, you'll find
nearly eighteen thousand entries between 1966 and 2010, some two-
thirds of which have been published within just the last decade.

Optimists portray this quest as an evolution in understanding, reduced stigma, and tolerance for different "learning styles." More jaundiced observers, however, see only a morass of medical ineptitude and corruption, gullible parents, and profiteering by pharmaceutical companies exploiting a lucrative new market in which an ordinary human variability is depicted as an illness, manageable only with a lifetime of pills. To me, it looks like a mix—just another variation on the combination of the heartwarming and the squalid that characterizes most of human history, with my own ancestors no exception.

MY SON BUZZ comes from a line of restless adventurers and escape artists. When I look back today with my new attention deficit lens, I recognize traits that seem to fit the profile as far back as his great-great-grandfather, a tailor by the name of Elias Eisenberg, who was born in the village of Drubnin, north of Warsaw. In 1898, my father's Grandpa Elya was the first member of our family to leave Eastern Europe, blazing a trail for other relatives by settling in Minneapolis with his wife and the first of what would be their eight children.

Five years later, in a voyage that lives on in family legend, Elias returned to Drubnin to retrieve his share of a family inheritance: a sum of 150,000 rubles, or about $6,000 today. All went well until his return to America, when he made an unscheduled stop in Monte Carlo, lingering for several months, as he feasted on caviar and champagne, consorted with a non-Jewish woman, and in a final grand gesture, tried to double his stake at the gambling table—and, naturally, lost it all.

Modern researchers have established that clinical-grade distraction often accompanies high-risk behavior, including drinking and gambling, encouraging me to wonder: was Buzz's great-great-grandfather a shtetl Fidgety Phil? Were his rash genes passed down to me and Buzz, like sharp-edged family jewels? Had Elya lacked those genetic *shpilkes*, Yiddish for "ants in his pants," might Buzz today be calmer, and maybe even a wealthy heir?

On the other hand, had his ancestor been less restless, might Buzz not have been born at all? After all, the same *shpilkes* that sent

Elias Eisenberg to Monte Carlo were probably also responsible for his leaving home just a few decades ahead of the Nazi Holocaust.

Following his European spree, Elias Eisenberg spent the rest of his life in obscurity in Minneapolis, quietly resuming his work as a tailor and his afternoon pinochle games. Yet from what I can tell, the episode had a lasting impact on at least one of his sons—Buzz's great-grandfather David, who grew up as stern and straitlaced as his father had been rambunctious. Alone among his siblings, he worked his way through college, continuing on to medical school and even volunteering for the navy. Circa 1917, he changed his surname to the less Jewish-sounding Ellison (a hidden tribute, since he meant "son of Elias"), in hopes it would help him rise through the ranks. He taught his three children to answer his commands with: "Aye, aye, sir!"

Determinedly different from his scamp of a father, my grandfather had two sons and a daughter of his own, all of whom followed him into medical careers in an especially busy era for doctors. On the heels of the global flu pandemic of 1918, which killed as many as 40 million people, came another, albeit less lethal plague, of *encephalitis lethargica,* the viral "sleepy sickness" that inflamed the brain, leaving many survivors permanently impaired. Afflicted children displayed dramatic changes in their behavior, becoming distracted and disobedient. In another milestone in the study of attention, researchers dubbed this syndrome "postencephalitic behavior disorder," making a clear link between brain physiology and the kind of behavior that was still widely blamed on bad character and upbringing. From this watershed streamed floods of other theories about potential physiological causes of major distraction, including birth trauma, head injuries, and exposure to lead, pesticides, and measles. Pediatricians started referring to the terribly restless children hauled into their clinics by wiped-out parents as having "minimal brain damage" or, later, "hyperkinetic impulse disorder."

Decades more would pass before scientists had the means to confirm George Still's early guess about family legacies. In the case of my father, however, it was already clear, as he grew up in Minneapolis in the late 1930s—fated as he was to a long, devoted marriage and a life of patient toil as an ear, nose, and throat doctor—that he had more in common with his restless grandfather than his name. A gifted student (who always waited until the eve of exams to study), he was also a locally notorious rascal, getting in scrapes with neighborhood kids and "taking girls out in canoes," as my Midwestern relatives have obliquely phrased it. His father blamed his mother for "spoiling" him, griping sarcastically that "Everybody's out of step except my son." Well into old age, however, my father continued to rebel within the confines of his mostly conventional life, distinguishing himself as a bon vivant, a budget-breaker, a bridge-burner, and a blurter of unwelcome truths.

"Understand your father!" my mother urged me, as a child.

More than forty years later, I'm still trying.

I WAS BORN IN Minneapolis in 1957, just two years after the Food and Drug Administration approved the sale of a new formula called Ritalin, containing the stimulant methylphenidate and initially prescribed to treat fatigue and depression. The chemist who concocted it for the Swiss pharmaceutical company Ciba-Geigy named the drug after his wife, Rita, certainly never guessing the fierce attacks it would provoke in a future when it would be prescribed to schoolchildren by the millions.

Shortly after my fourth birthday, my father followed an impulse nearly as bold as his grandfather's flight from Poland. Later he would tell us that he'd fallen in love with the San Francisco Bay Area while stationed as a wartime medic at the Letterman Army Medical Center. So intent was he on returning, apparently, that he ignored the protests of his wife, sister, and ageing parents to move his family from Minneapolis to the West Coast, where he joined a new medical practice. From what I could tell as I grew up, however, the move didn't make him happy, or our home particularly peaceful. If my own genes inclined me to restlessness, the frequent dinner-table arguments between my father and my brothers, linked forever in my mind with tuna melts and TV reports on the Vietnam War, made me positively jumpy.

School offered little refuge. The long hours in the classroom were at least as torturous for me as they are today for Buzz. Early on, my teachers complained that I was underperforming, and I often got sent to the principal's office for passing notes and talking back. By sixth grade, bored and daydreaming, I'd devised a diversionary tactic for when I got caught spacing out—I abbreviated it as AQQ for "ask a question, quick!" and it has served me well into adulthood. But no one, back then, ever suggested there was anything clinically wrong. It took a lot in the 1970s for a kid to be sent to a shrink, and girls, in particular, often slipped under the radar. Even today, various studies show boys are at least three times more likely to be diagnosed with ADD, despite experts' belief that this exaggerates the true prevalence of the disorder, which they say is only somewhat more common in boys than girls. In girls, still so much more rigorously trained to play nice, the problem more often surfaces as something else—something internally rather than externally harmful—such as depression, drug abuse, or an eating disorder. Experts say about one-third of all people diagnosed with ADD develop an anxiety disorder, a statistic that doesn't surprise me.

By the time I was twelve, Buzz's age today, I was just as rebellious, although usually more covertly so. I regularly lied to my parents, hitchhiked, shoplifted, sneaked out to see a creepy older guy I met on the bus, memorized passages of the Yippie outlaw Abbie Hoffman's *Steal This Book,* and constantly plotted my getaway. When my eighth-grade English teacher wasn't watching, I penned neat, cursive letters on binder paper: "I read about your commune in *Steal This Book,*" I informed a "cybernated-tribal society" in Oregon. "Do you like visitors? Would you accept new members?"

No one, perhaps fortunately, ever answered these inquiries. Yet in time, I finagled at least a minor escape: out of the high school where I'd earned a reputation as a screwup in my first year. I transferred to another school, ostensibly because I wanted to take Latin, and there abruptly turned a new leaf: joining the tennis team, becoming editor of the school paper, and getting a national award for my score on a college entry test. Inspired by my diligent older sister and brothers, and uplifted by two extraordinary English teachers, I began to study hard, cultivating a steely will to compensate for a flickering mind. By the time I squeaked into Stanford University in 1975, I'd also chosen my future career—motivated, like so many budding journalists of the time, by the rebellious achievements of Woodward and Bernstein, I. F. Stone, and the Italian interviewer Oriana Fallaci.

I was still rebelling, too—at least within my family's context. While all three of my siblings were bound for medical school, like our father, and his father, I'd decided to become a foreign correspondent, running away from home in the socially sanctioned way.

Seen again through that ADD lens, my career choice is hardly surprising. Newspapers have long been magnets for restless, impatient people. The urgency of deadlines, forcing us to put all other options aside; the faraway adventures; the constant conflicts; the opportunities to tweak the noses of those in charge—all wrapped up in the daily mission to deliver novelty to other novelty-seekers—make them irresistible for people like me. Flying into disaster zones in the 1980s and 1990s—the Mexico City earthquake, the death-squad violence in El Salvador, the U.S. invasion of Panama, the terrorist bombing of the Buenos Aires Jewish community center—turned up the volume and contrast of daily life. Who needs Ritalin when you can cover coups?

I GOT MY FIRST full-time job in 1981, covering local beats for the *San Jose Mercury News*. As I'd only later learn, this was just one year after another milestone in the annals of clinical-grade distraction: the christening of the syndrome as "attention deficit disorder" in the psychiatric atlas, the *Diagnostic and Statistical Manual*. The new name reflected a newly compassionate focus on the interior life of the afflicted, a perspective originally proposed by the Canadian psychologist Virginia Douglas.

I was still a toddler when Douglas began working with seriously distracted children at an outpatient clinic at the Montreal Children's Hospital. She was struck by how many of the kids (mostly boys) couldn't seem to control their impulses. Easily bored, they rushed through their schoolwork, making careless mistakes, cursing, and squabbling. When she gave one boy a hug, he slapped her on her butt.

Douglas was equally charmed and alarmed, as she told me, half a century later. "You couldn't help loving them," she said. "They were so forthright and so genuine often in telling you exactly what they thought. They didn't have all those inhibitions, and there was something refreshing and lovely about that. You wished you could get away with a lot of what they did."

Douglas's new paradigm—that the impulsive behavior was rooted in a problem in sustaining attention—would ultimately contribute to a significant expansion in the number of children eligible for diagnosis and treatment through the 1980s. And while this trend raised huge controversy, it all but escaped my notice at the time, engrossed as I was with first building up, and then trying to piece back together my new career. Assigned to the courts and cops beat at the *Mercury News*, I'd produced a series of dramatic front-page stories, which unfortunately included several boneheaded mistakes: errors in reporting numbers, names, and other details. Each of the requisite published corrections brought me that same, awful, ice-water-down-my-back feeling as I felt when I took Cliff Saron's test. *Nope, that couldn't have been me! No way I did that.*

I'll always be grateful, as well as slightly mystified, that my editors never fired me, even after the terrible afternoon in July of 1981 when an error I made in a high-profile, death-penalty murder case prompted the $11 million lawsuit. At that point, however, they did suspend me for a couple of days, gently suggesting I use the time to seek professional help. That's when I found Dr. Y., a bearded Irishman with a warm smile and wild laugh, who because he was still in training offered semitraditional Freudian therapy at a discount. I lay on his couch and rambled away, three or four times a week. As was the norm then, we chalked up my self-destructive behavior and snake's-belly-level self-esteem to my parents' errors. I stayed angry at my father, in particular, for many more years.

At the *Mercury News*, meanwhile, I sought more practical advice from the paper's star investigative reporter, Pete Carey, who was kind enough to tell me he'd also made some errors in his past. The term "ADD" still wasn't in wide use, but the word in the newsroom was that Carey was one of those seriously distracted geniuses—"stuck on input," as he himself once described it—until deadlines forced him to produce. He seemed to understand my predicament, and urged me to work on slowing down and sharpening my focus. "You just have to eyeball every word," he said.

I had enough ambition to work that hard, and harder. Keeping in mind my new eyeball mantra, I resolved to win back my editors' respect by showing them what I could do as a foreign correspondent, on my own time and my own dime. I spent my next few vacations from the courts and cops beat reporting freelance stories from war zones in Central America.

By the end of 1983, when I was twenty-five years old, I'd redeemed my reputation sufficiently to be assigned to a story that, to the surprise of almost everyone involved, would help change the course of history in the faraway Philippines. The country had burst into the news after opposition activist Benigno Aquino was gunned down on the airport tarmac in Manila, with the obvious involvement of the U.S.-backed dictatorship of Ferdinand and Imelda Marcos. As protests increased in Manila and reverberated among the thousands of Filipinos living in the San Francisco Bay Area, my editors assigned Carey and me to track down clues that the notoriously corrupt rulers and their cronies were siphoning off tens of millions of dollars from U.S. aid and using it to buy U.S. real estate.

The paper's Tokyo bureau chief, Lew Simons, sent us investigative leads from Filipino opposition groups in the Philippines, and Carey and I spent six months gathering others and chasing them down. We worked late into the evenings, leaning over the paper's mammoth Coyote computer terminals. We argued so often over who'd do what next that a colleague started calling us "the Bickersons." Yet we saved most of our outrage for the Marcoses' cynical thievery, as we systematically exposed their network of phony corporations to buy land and buildings from San Francisco to Manhattan.

Our series, published in 1985, inspired a U.S. congressional investigation and raised such ire in the Philippines that it forced Ferdinand Marcos to call early elections, which, to his surprise, he lost. I flew in and out of Manila for several months to cover these developments, even running through the chaos of Malacanang Palace with hundreds of Filipino celebrants the night the Marcoses fled for Hawaii. The series won a Pulitzer Prize the following year, and one year later my editors finally assigned me to a foreign beat, as chief of the paper's bureau in Mexico City. It looked as if all of my dreams were coming true.

"Millions of Mexicans are trying to come here, and you're going in the opposite direction!" my father complained, which I only much later understood was his way of saying he'd miss me. I stayed in Mexico for the next six years, after which I jumped ship to the *Miami Herald,* which assigned me to Rio de Janeiro.

While covering my new beat—the southern half of South America—I tracked events in six countries, hopped planes on short notice, and conducted interviews in Spanish while taking notes in English and conversing with colleagues in Portuguese. I married Jack, then a freelance journalist, whom I'd met in Nicaragua, in 1990, and gave birth to Buzz and Max during our years in Rio, juggling my motherly duties with the help of a nanny, a cook, and an office assistant. I covered fast-paced stories involving wars, coups, soccer matches, samba parades, currency speculation, drug-trafficking, child labor, and Amazon deforestation, never missing a flight or a deadline. (*Does it count if you delay them until the last minute, while your editors are pulling out their hair?*) The worst price my offbeat behavior exacted during these years, at least as best I can recall, was the loss of the *Herald'*s longtime Rio office assistant, Marilene, who quit in a huff, complaining about my habit of running into her office with pieces of recycled paper on which I'd written some new thing I wanted her to do. "*Those leetle beets of paper!*" were her furious last words.

I had no idea back then what a lark it all was, attention-wise, compared to what awaited when I settled back home. I had yet to appreciate how well suited my brain was for the short-term, exhilarating sprints required for deadline reporting, and what a struggle it would be to adapt to the day-in, day-out marathon of generally unassisted stay-at-home mothering of two high-maintenance boys.

MY SON BUZZ, as I've mentioned, seemed just fine during the first years of our transition to the Northern California suburbs. He got invited to lots of birthday parties and did well in school—right up until second grade, when his teacher started calling to complain about how he was tuning out in class. "He goes to the beach!" she'd tell me repeatedly, sometimes even saying it in front of Buzz. His previously positive attitude soon changed. By the end of that year, he was frequently pretending to be sick, fighting me to stay home. "Mom, why don't you homeschool me?" he pleaded. *Maybe, if I'd been a better mother, I'd have done that.*

Buzz's grade school principal was the first to speculate that he might have attention deficit disorder, an idea I hadn't previously considered. I'd been wondering if Buzz were getting enough sleep, hovering over him at night to check his breathing. But the principal encouraged me to have Buzz checked by a psychologist, resulting in what would be the first of a long round of appointments with medical, psychological, and educational professionals.

I ended up going to all but a few of them alone, or with Buzz, reporting back in the evening to Jack. The happy-go-lucky freelancer with whom I'd traveled the world for more than a decade before we had kids was by now commuting to a job as an editor of foreign news at the *San Francisco Chronicle,* which, like other newspapers throughout the country, had become a grim and stressful place. Together with his colleagues lucky enough to still have a job, Jack was situationally distracted: working longer, irregular hours to fill in for a decimated staff. Added to which Jack has never been a particularly avid therapy buff. Nor did he even seem to notice most of the troubles with Buzz, which by then were keeping me awake at night. He supported my decision to seek professional help but mostly stayed on the sidelines.

Buzz's pediatrician recommended a psychiatrist who was covered by our insurance: a short man in his late sixties, with a hoarse voice. The clock on his wall said "Strattera," while his pen said "Concerta," both names of pharmaceutical treatments for ADD. After less than twenty minutes of conversation, he recommended—*surprise, surprise!*—that Buzz start medication. "We have many decades of experience with these drugs," he assured me. "They are very well tolerated and very effective. We'd know by now if they weren't safe."

I was still doubtful, as he could probably tell by the way I was vigorously shaking my head. I'm not a fan of quick fixes, at least not where developing brains are concerned. I'm just not that kind of mom; I'm more of an I-turned-down-the-epidural-*twice* mom, an at-least-mostly stay-at-home mom, a Suzuki violin and listen-to-Raffi-till-you-puke mom. Put my kid on *speed*? Please. Tuned into the news as both Jack and I were, we were well aware of the growing popular backlash against medicating kids. Googling away, I'd learned about all the potential side effects, including facial tics, high blood pressure, insomnia, weight loss, and stunted growth—the growth issue being particularly discouraging, since Buzz was already the shortest kid in his class. At night, I'd been reading aloud to Jack from *Talking Back to Ritalin*, in which the rebel psychiatrist Dr. Peter Breggin warns that prescription stimulants turn children into "zombies." The drugs "make good caged animals," Dr. Breggin has said.

"We'd really rather not start Buzz on meds," I told Dr. Concerta Pen, still shaking my head. "Aren't there other options?"

He shook his head back at me. Resistance at this point was risky, he warned, adding: "A lot of these kids self-medicate, and end up abusing drugs."

I shrugged, not sure I believed him, and he shot me a sorrowful smile, as if to say: *Another granola-munching loser, ruining her son's life.*

Back home, I plunged back into Googling, ordering more books, and setting up appointments for Buzz to see other therapists who weren't covered by our insurance but who seemed to have more time for more time-consuming approaches. For nine months in 2005, when Buzz was nine years old and in fourth grade, he and I also attended an experimental, weekly, parent-and-child behavior modification course offered for free by researchers at the University of California in San Francisco. It was there that on the basis of tests and lengthy interviews, Buzz was for the first time formally diagnosed with both attention deficit disorder and oppositional defiant disorder. The researchers also taught me to keep complicated charts with stickers and smiley faces to track points earned by behaviors such as getting out of bed on time, going to school without staging a revolt, and remembering and completing homework assignments.

Trying to be fair, I also maintained charts for Max, then six, but while he earnestly racked up points, Buzz poured his energy into breaking the new rules and throwing tantrums when Max got rewarded. My other problem was that while all the other parents showed up with neat, computer-generated reward charts, mine were scrawled freehand on copy paper with old drafts of magazine stories on the other side, while I kept changing the reward categories, like an airline on the verge of bankruptcy. I didn't pass my charts around the table, like the other parents did. Yet I was also growing sadly convinced that even if I'd had charts to die for—with fanciful fonts, rainbow colors, and smiley faces galore—it wouldn't really have helped.

By Buzz's fifth-grade year, my boys were home all the time. After losing his own friends, Buzz had scared off the last of Max's friends who'd dared to come over for playdates. Both of them balked at after-school sports or even playing outdoors, begging instead to watch TV or play computer games, and tumbling through the house like squirrels, knocking each other's head against the furniture, making hash out of my increasingly weak attempts to concentrate on anything else.

"BORRRRRRRRN FREE!" Max would yodel, after sneaking up behind my back. No one ever suggested Max had a disorder; he was just extremely intense. Sitting at the kitchen table with his daily PB&J, he'd scat-sing—Louis Armstrong doing "Rockin' Robin"—in between scattershot questions ("Will the continents ever merge again to form Pangaea?" "What's seven times three?" "Did Frida Kahlo really have a mustache?" "Is your career still 'in the toilet'?") until, cognitively whipsawed, I'd burn the rice or drop a fork down the disposal. Then I'd laugh. But Buzz never laughed. Every high-pitched squeal of Max's, every clever observation, song, or siren impression ("AhOOOGAH!!") was for Buzz the most personal of insults, often ending in a double-death-grip on the floor. Max perfected a piteous cry for such occasions, efficiently triggering my most primitive maternal rage.

Whatever hopes Jack and I might have had for a social life during this time, or I might have had of paying serious attention to my work, were thwarted as a procession of temporary babysitters quit on us. There was a friend's teenaged son who came over to play with the kids for a few bucks while I was trying to meet a deadline, but who crept to my shed window within the first hour of brotherly combat and whispered, "Just shoot me!" Then the initially enthusiastic eighth-grade neighborhood girl who mysteriously got busy with homework after the first shift. And the pretty blond community college student who stayed through a dinner hour while Jack and I snuck off to a movie, but left in tears the minute we came home, mumbling something about a squirt gun. And the stout Jehovah's Witness, sent from the expensive agency I'd turned to in despair, who read magazines while my sons punched each other, devoured entire packages of cookies, and played video games for three hours.

But at last came a temp who was unlike all the others. A bald-headed Buddhist, with a beatific smile, this sitter, whom I'll call Stu, was referred by my niece, who had dated him briefly. He arrived at our door like a soulful Mary Poppins, in that season of despair, and went right to work charming the boys, even getting them outside, and telling me all about Eckhart Tolle during long conversations in our kitchen, as I made snacks for them, silently praying he'd never leave. For a few, golden weeks, he did keep returning, at $20 an hour plus gas, and even taught the boys to meditate, which they seemed to enjoy mostly for the chance to play with the incense and matches. But then Stu vanished as abruptly as he'd arrived, quitting school to embark on a live-in-the-moment road trip with a friend. The boys and I still miss him.

Aside from that blissful interlude, I didn't get much writing done during Buzz's pre-adolescence, and by night I began to have a recurring dream. I was a foreign correspondent again, off on assignment, spending lots of money, but for some reason not filing any stories. I realized my editors were about to catch on and fire me, but I couldn't sit down to write. Apparently, I was stuck on input.

And then life handed me another major distraction: a series of migraines, which grew so intense over the course of several months that I ended up in the hospital ER a couple times, begging for morphine. While at first I chalked up the headaches to the normal toll of motherhood, a brain scan finally revealed that I had a slow-growing "benign" tumor called a meningioma. What a blessing that it wasn't one of those nightmare diagnoses, like a life-threatening glioblastoma or astrocytoma! On the other hand, I still needed surgery—*brain surgery.* And while the doctor said I could put it off for a year, it was a year that I therefore spent additionally preoccupied, even as Jack and I took care to keep the details from the kids.

With my own parents and siblings, I indulged in our family's traditional coping trick: black humor. At dinners at my parents' house, my brother David, himself a surgeon, would sneak up on me and make loud, buzz-saw noises behind my head. My other brother, Jim, a psychiatrist and avid prankster, mailed me an invitation he'd printed up to join a phony group he called the "Elective Fontanelle Association." The card had an image of a rainbow rising out of a hole in a person's head, with the motto "Open to experience . . ." In time, I even managed to joke with Buzz and Max, telling them about the brain surgery patient who when asked if he'd do it again, asks, "Do *what* again?"

We all kept making jokes right up to the eve of the surgery, when, once the boys were asleep, I snuck out to my shed for a few moments to write provisionary good-bye notes, weeping as I left them under a book on my desk. But all went well, and I recovered just fine, reveling in my new lease on life—and no more migraines!—for three lovely months. Then, during a routine exam, my internist found some bumps on my throat that turned out to be thyroid cancer. I had to have another surgery, this time right away. Once again, however, I was lucky, and fine, and by that autumn back into my routine of trying to work and running errands, when, while dashing along on my bike to an event at Max's school, with his violin poised on the handlebars, I braked too suddenly and fell right over, fracturing both my arms.

During the long wait in the emergency room, I could no longer escape the feeling that the Universe was trying to tell me something. But what? And why did it have to be so nasty about it? Especially when it came to Buzz, who had to choose *this* time to become extra difficult. In the close-quarters late afternoons after school, he refused to help out or even take care of himself, adamantly resisting doing any homework, brushing his teeth, or picking up his clothes from the floor. Everything that should have been routine became a major battle. *How can he be so angry with me? Doesn't he see how I'm suffering?*

The harder it was for me to focus on him, the more he fought for my attention. On one afternoon when I'd promised to play Monopoly but could hardly open my eyes, much less get out of bed, he stood in front of me, demanding, "Can't you take another pill?" And then, "Couldn't you just play cards then? You could just sit there with the cards in your hand!" And finally, in a stern, parental tone: "Mom, I'm *very disappointed in you.*"

My year of migraines was my worst year with him, but once they stopped, we managed to find at least one refuge we could share. I'd become a fan of meditation in the weeks leading up to my brain surgery, after discovering that focusing on my breath on sleepless nights helped stave off panic attacks, and had begun attending classes at Spirit Rock, a Buddhist retreat perched in the hills amid the ranchlands about a half hour's drive from our home. The center offered a special class for middle school students, and Buzz, to my surprise, agreed to attend. Maybe it was due to all those happy memories of burning incense with our fugitive Buddhist babysitter, but he seemed at home right away, especially enjoying the frantic games of "Dharma-tag," the center's clever, get-your-ya-yas-out prelude to sitting in silence. While waiting for him, I'd sometimes walk up the starlit path to the center's main hall and sit in silence, by myself. It felt so good that I started pitching freelance stories on the subject, so I could learn more.

This was the contemplative trail that led to Cliff Saron's windy research refuge in the Rockies, where I confided in him about all my fights with Buzz, including that time on the highway when I yelled "Shut up!"

"That should *never* happen," Saron said.

Yeah, easy for *him* to say, I thought, relieved, at least, that I hadn't mentioned all the other things I'd yelled. Still, I agreed with him, at heart, and was already wondering: *How can I get there? To that place of inner calm and self-restraint where that kind of thing* never *happens?*

CHAPTER 2

EMERGENCY

Crossing Lines in the Ritalin Wars

What is the pill that will keep us well,
serene, contented?

HENRY DAVID THOREAU

ON A WINTRY AFTERNOON DURING BUZZ'S SIXTH-GRADE YEAR,
I was frying latkes with my friend Sally when she told me how her
husband had persuaded her to start their son on stimulants.

Wow, I thought. *Their kid's a little dreamy, but he couldn't be caus-*
ing half of the trouble we've had with Buzz.

"Phil says he's sick of being harassed by Mark's teachers," Sally
told me, jabbing at the oily potatoes with a paper towel. "Mark spaces
out all the time in class, and the few times he actually does his
homework, he loses it before he can turn it in."

After just two weeks on meds, Mark's teachers seemed happier,
Sally acknowledged. Yet her son was losing weight, and he had already
been too skinny, and what other harm might the drugs be doing?

Nearly eighteen months had passed since my appointment with
the doctor who had urged us to start Buzz on stimulants—months in
which I'd spent scores of hours and several thousand dollars seeking
alternatives. My main coup had been to track down a well-reviewed
child psychiatrist, Dr. Z., who wasn't covered by our insurance, had an
office an hour's drive away from our house, took fourteen months

before he had a free appointment, and charged $150 an hour for talk therapy. Buzz had also started sessions with an after-school tutor I'll call Blossom, a reputed miracle worker who charged $65 an hour with a mandatory minimum of two hours a week, but who was already winning Buzz over with her merry jokes and practice of doling out gumballs along with the study-skills training. On many of the other afternoons, I was hauling Buzz around, almost always against his will, trying, and repeatedly failing, to interest him in some widely recommended, obviously essential, structure-providing/character-building after-school activity: we tried, in succession, baseball practice, a swim team, tennis lessons, martial arts, and fencing, in addition to his now mandatory, twice-a-week Hebrew school, since in just two years he was going to be ready for his bar mitzvah ceremony. (Was he overscheduled? Underscheduled? I know I was overscheduled. . . .)

I wondered if Phil knew about all the promising alternatives to drugs. A few hours later, I spotted him at the Hanukah party where Sally and I had brought our plates of latkes. He was sitting near a wall decorated with silver tinsel, munching a dreidel-shaped cookie, and tapping his foot to the wail of a klezmer clarinet. *Not a care in the world.*

I walked over, gave him a friendly hug, and pulled up a chair to ask if he'd ever heard of Dr. Peter Breggin. No? I'd be happy to lend him my copy of *Talking Back to Ritalin*. Had he heard the recent news about how Canada had taken the amphetamine Adderall off the market after it gave kids *heart attacks*? Or the reports linking stimulants to depression, as well as potential chromosome damage— i.e., a precursor for cancer?

Phil peered at me with an incredulous look that I somehow managed to ignore. I was, after all, on a roll.

Didn't Phil agree that the real problem behind this supposed epidemic of attention deficit disorder was with our failed educational system? Had he ever even questioned the teachers who'd bullied him into this? Couldn't he see he was getting his kid hooked on *speed*?

"This is really none of your business," he told me.

Huh? Hey, couldn't he see I was just trying to help?

. . .

AT THIS WRITING, a reported 2.5 million U.S. children are taking medication for attention deficit disorder. Most often they take stimulants, chiefly methylphenidate, the active ingredient in Ritalin.

The practice dates from a remarkable accident that took place in the 1930s, at a Rhode Island institute that was conducting research on children with brain disorders. The pediatrician Charles Bradley and his staff had been using a primitive X-ray device known as a pneumoencephalogram to study children whose complaints ranged from epilepsy to autism to the mysterious restlessness then referred to by that catchy phrase "hyperkinetic impulse disorder."

People who've had MRI brain scans often complain about the noise and discomfort of lying for as long as an hour inside a metal tube. They have no idea how lucky they are to have escaped the pneumoencephalogram, a precursor that required a patient to have air injected into his spinal column and then be rotated about in a specially designed chair. The torturous procedure gave many of the children nausea and intense headaches, which the researchers treated with Benzedrine, a prescription decongestant and amphetamine. And, presto! Suddenly the children were behaving like little angels—angels who, to the researchers' added delight, were also turning in much better math homework. Bradley's reports on this phenomenon led to Benzedrine becoming known as "the arithmetic pill."

And wasn't that a paradox? A stimulant was helping hyperactive kids sit still. You'd think it would send them into overdrive, but as Bradley discovered, the medication instead improved their focus and self-control. That led to his educated guess that the drug must be somehow strengthening the children's sluggish inhibitory system: those weak brakes on the brain.

That's still the basic theory today. While modern neuroscientists acknowledge they still don't know precisely how the stimulants work, they believe that the medication, just like coffee and cocaine, increases the brain's ability to use dopamine and other key neurotransmitters, the chemical messengers flowing between the synapses, the gaps between brain cells.

Bradley's experiments took place at the dawn of serious interest in using drugs to treat psychiatric complaints, a trend that has brought the incontestable advantage of greatly reducing harsher treatments, such as lobotomies, locked wards, and electroshock. By the 1960s, millions of Americans were being treated with drugs such as chlorpromazine, marketed as Thorazine, for schizophrenia. And one decade later, lithium was approved for bipolar disorder, and methylphenidate, marketed as Ritalin, was on the way to becoming the favored treatment for seriously distracted children. Similar drugs aimed at curbing distraction soon joined a rapidly expanding market, which nearly tripled in size worldwide between 1993 and 2007.

At this writing, America remains the world's unmatched leader in stimulant consumption, with an estimated one in twenty-five U.S. children and adolescents taking ADD drugs. This is part of a broader phenomenon: Americans spent $291 billion on prescription drugs in 2008, with nearly 65 percent of us, and increasingly also our cats and dogs, taking one or more medications every day. Our energetic capitalist system is undoubtedly a factor: the United States and New Zealand are the world's only two nations that allow prescription drugmakers to market their products directly to consumers, in magazines and on TV, and those ads surely seem to boost sales. U.S. doctors, on average, are also quicker to diagnose, and treat, an attention disorder than colleagues in other countries. U.S. children are three times more likely to be treated with stimulants than are children, for instance, in the Netherlands and Germany.

Stimulant sales have nonetheless been rapidly growing in Europe and elsewhere, for the simple reason that no other treatment has been found to be as efficient in calming those jitters and keeping kids on task. This effect, witnessed by doctors for years, was resoundingly confirmed in 1999, in the first published results from the $12 million Multimodal Treatment Study of Children with Attention Deficit Hyperactivity Disorder, known as the MTA. Medication proved better than behavior therapy for seriously distracted children, as this landmark study reported—and almost as good as a combination of the two.

Most American parents with diagnosed kids have heeded this guidance, as delivered by their family doctors. In recent years, nearly 60 percent of U.S. kids diagnosed with attention deficit disorder have been treated with medication. The trend owes much to both history and economics. The boom years for pediatric stimulants—the 1970s through the 1990s—coincided with the dramatic migration of mothers into the workforce, a rise in divorce rates, and a general squeezing of the middle class. Today, more than half of U.S. families are earning less than the so-called living wage, recently estimated at $14 an hour. With all that juggling and belt-tightening and stress, how many parents have had the money or mental bandwidth to explore time-consuming, costly alternative treatments? And, of course, why would they want to, with doctors and prestigious experts on TV so bullish about the medications?

In the year 2000, one year after the first MTA findings were reported, Dr. Harold Koplewicz, vice chairman of the New York University Child Study Center, suggested, on *Good Morning America,* that doctors and teachers would be justified in reporting parents to Child Protective Services for refusing to medicate a diagnosed child.

In other words, *not* putting your scatterbrained child on speed could amount to child abuse.

This probably made sense for some families. Yet Koplewicz's aggressive stance surely helped fuel the mounting backlash that became known as the Ritalin Wars. By the late 1990s, especially in well-educated, upwardly mobile, bicoastal U.S. communities, arguments like the one I had with Phil were becoming common. More than a dozen U.S. states were either contemplating or had passed resolutions banning teachers from even talking to parents about pharmaceutical approaches to ADD, while plaintiffs' lawyers filed half a dozen class-action suits against psychiatrists and drug manufacturers. By 2003, however, these suits had all been dismissed, and the pro-stimulant forces were prevailing where it counted: in doctor's offices, and in homes and schools.

I STAYED ON the anti-med warpath through the spring of 2007, even as Buzz took a definite turn for the worse. By then, he was fighting every morning against going to school, even missing the bus on purpose, obliging me to drive him and then, often, push him out the car door. "I hate you!" he'd yell at me, day after day.

How in the world had we reached this point? I could so easily remember when motherhood seemed like the high point of my life, when I was energized rather than depleted by signs of Buzz's take-no-prisoners-will. Pacing the floor for an hour at a time with my yowling infant, I'd picture myself as Menelaus, in that scene from the *Odyssey* where he wrestles the sea god who morphs from a lion to a serpent to a leopard, to finally—asleep at last!—a flowering tree. The trick was to keep holding on, and I did. Hemingway, keep your bulls and big fish! This was true life-or-death drama, giving my life an exhilarating new focus.

Barely a decade later, however, I was no longer the brave heroine, and I often wondered how much longer I'd be able to hold on. By that awful spring, Buzz had not a single close friend, nor any interest to engage his lively mind, besides TV and Game Boy, and his ever-more-elaborate visions of the costly gifts I should buy him. Jack and I shuddered at these portents of values so determinedly opposed to our bean-eating, Prius-driving, debt-averse lifestyle. Were we nurturing the next Donald Trump?

At home, he was constantly in a rage: swearing, throwing shoes, banging his head against the wall. I felt terrible for him, but worse for myself, drawn back to the worst nights of my own childhood, with that old, breathless tightening of panic in my chest, wanting nothing more than to run away from home.

After hours of being railed at by Buzz, I'd pick a fight with Jack the minute he walked in the door from work, a passing-a-slap-down-

the-line routine that as he wittily observed came straight from the
Three Stooges.

"Do you think the sofa needs to be cleaned?" he might innocently
ask.

"Why are you asking me? Why don't *you* take charge of something around here for a change? And why don't you start acting like a
parent, while you're at it?" I'd snarl. I was already aware of the reports announcing that mothers and fathers of clinically distracted
children are more than twice as likely to separate or divorce. *But why
did I already feel so alone?*

Back then, it seemed like every time I turned around, I'd see
Buzz gulping down another one of those super-sized "energy drinks"
in vogue at his middle school—the ones with names like "Red Bull,"
"Monster," and "Rock Star." He'd buy them with money he said
he'd "found," or sometimes I'd give in to his begging and buy them
for him. I recalled the Concerta-pen doc's warning that without
pharmaceutical support, Buzz would "self-medicate," and fretted over
the cumulative effect of all that unregulated caffeine, taurine, gua-
rana, and God-knows-what-else. *Maybe Ritalin was the more heart-
healthy choice!*

Other parents—those well-rested, youthful looking, skiing and
bowling and yucking-it-up-with-their-kids other parents I'd see around
the elementary school—by then were clearly avoiding me. I suspected that if Buzz had autism, God forbid, or even a leg in a cast, I'd
have more friends. But here was a kid who seemed normal, even unusually bright, when he wasn't behaving atrociously. Why wouldn't
they blame his lazy, incompetent mom? I sure would have.

By April of that year, my afternoon telephone rants to my mother
had reached such a pitch that she sent an SOS to her brother, a child
psychiatrist (our family is full of them) in Los Angeles. On a Sunday
afternoon, Jack and I gave the boys an extra hour of Game Boy while
we talked to Uncle David on the phone. After listening patiently to
everything we had to say, he quietly told us that it was "imperative" to
start Buzz on meds. He also cited the MTA's conclusions that the
stimulants were effective and safe.

I trusted my uncle. *But could I trust the MTA?*

Even as that landmark study was wholly government-funded, most of its prestigious researchers were simultaneously serving as paid consultants for and/or getting research grants from manufacturers of attention deficit disorder drugs, including Novartis, Shire, McNeil Pediatrics, and Eli Lilly. Why shouldn't I assume that the money that supported their careers influenced the kinds of questions they asked and the conclusions they drew? In 2006, the same year in which I was trying to figure out whom I could trust, the *Washington Post* revealed that every single expert involved in writing criteria for psychiatry's bible, the *Diagnostic and Statistical Manual,* had ties to companies selling drugs for the relevant ailments. Among leading ADD experts, Harvard's internationally respected Dr. Joseph Biederman was a paid adviser to six drug companies, a paid speaker for six companies, and a paid researcher for ten companies, while the equally influential investigator and popular author Dr. Russell Barkley earned nearly a quarter of his 2007 income from ADD drug manufacturers. Dr. Edward Hallowell, who touted methylphenidate in his popular books, was a paid consultant for McNeil Pediatrics, manufacturer of the long-acting formula called Concerta.

I'd been conditioned, as a journalist, to mock such compromised sources. Yet the crisis with Buzz persuaded me to keep an open mind. And as I continued to read and ask questions, I came to wonder if the researcher/consultants were in fact correct in arguing that the meds really weren't as toxic as they'd been described in all those scary news stories I'd cited in my argument with Phil.

The alarm about heart attacks, as I discovered, was based on a federal government probe of just eleven reported deaths between 1992 and 2005, in which all of the children involved had preexisting heart conditions. The study linking stimulants with depression was also problematic, in that researchers had *injected* rats with methylphenidate, a procedure quite different from having children swallow it, as prescribed. (Not only were the doses relatively higher, but injecting the drug brings on a faster, addictive rush.) The cancer concern turned out to be based on a small, preliminary study by a group of University of Texas scientists, whose findings, as I learned, were refuted by U.S. federal investigators.

Not all of the downsides had been overplayed. Researchers had solidly confirmed, for instance, that the stimulants stunt growth—by a not-insignificant average of about three-fourths of an inch after three years—on top of other worrisome potential side effects, such as raised blood pressure, insomnia, and tics. But were even these enough to rule out the meds altogether? For a week after talking with my uncle, I loitered anxiously in the no-man's-land between the purportedly profiteering pill-pushers and the mixed bag of anti-drug crusaders—Scientologists, allergists, chiropractors, and nutritionists—all equally eager to exploit my worst fears. I felt like Dorothy in that scene from *The Wizard of Oz* in which the Scarecrow instructs her to proceed in two different directions at once.

But then came another of those endless, after-school late afternoons, when Buzz and I were fighting again, for a reason I no longer remember. The part that I'll never forget is when he ran into the kitchen, grabbed a butcher knife, waved it at me, and then held it against his own throat.

He was saying something I couldn't hear over of the sound of someone screaming.

Hold on, that was me *screaming.*

"STOP!"

"STOP!"

"STOP!"

Could this get any worse? By then, what scared me so much more than Buzz's anger was my own—particularly when he seemed to threaten Max's safety. I'd grabbed him and shaken him on several occasions by then, always to my anguished remorse. Later I'd learn that clinically distracted children are significantly more likely than peers to be physically harmed by their frustrated parents. A minority of other parents end up shipping their unmanageable offspring off to wilderness programs or boarding schools. I never imagined I could join them. I always thought that I had one of those magical mother's hearts, which would keep on thumping, no matter what. And yet by this time

I'd already, and more than once, brandished the nuclear bomb of parenting. "There are places," I'd told Buzz. "Military school. Boarding school. The point is this just can't continue. You. May. Not. Destroy. This. Family."

As I watched my desperate son wave that big knife, however, I felt my heart thumping again. Buzz noticed the tears in my eyes and joined with me, crying. He dropped the knife, as Max, also weeping, ran in from his room. I wrapped my arms around them both, as, ashes, ashes, we sank to the floor.

Stop. *Stop.* How could I make it stop?

BY NOW, it's probably clear where this is leading.

About three weeks after the knife incident, Jack and I stood shoulder-to-shoulder in our kitchen, confronting our first-born child as he chewed on a mango-jalapeño sausage.

It was a gray morning in early May, just a few minutes before Buzz needed to catch his bus to school. The fog had finally rolled in from the bay, squelching a week-long heat wave. But the air was hazy, no doubt loaded with particulate matter from coal-burning power plants in China.

Jack and I had rehearsed what came next. I held out my hand to display a barrel-shaped pill, about the size and color of a child's unbrushed tooth: an 18 mg. dose of the long-acting stimulant pill Concerta.

Jack had agreed to do the talking. His eyes were fixed on Buzz, and he was speaking faster than usual.

"Buzz, you know we've discussed trying out medication to help you, and we're going to do that today," he said.

Buzz looked up at us as if it were the first he'd heard of this, even though we had been working up to it by then for several days. Swamped with despair, I considered, again, how different things would be if, say, Buzz's meltdowns were due to an overactive thyroid. Were that the case, we wouldn't think twice about addressing the biological source of his troubles. But because the problem is inside

Buzz's brain instead of his glands, this was much more than a medical decision. It was instead a moral, cultural, and political choice, which we and millions of other parents are usually forced to make in the midst of a crisis, and while ducking a hailstorm of contradictory data.

There are no easy answers, only a painful weighing and re-weighing of ultimately unmeasurable risks. One woman I'd later interview, describing her own tortured decision following escalating conflicts with her son, told me how her mother-in-law had scolded her about the possible impact on her son's height.

"Better short than dead," this resolute mother retorted.

"We're going to try this," Jack told Buzz at our kitchen table. "If it doesn't help, we'll stop, but we're going to try, because we think it may."

Buzz shook his head no. I kept my hand out, my eyes on his. The pill was in the center of my palm, a bitter cocktail on a butler's tray.

Jack and I were bluffing, of course. We weren't prepared to shove the pill past Buzz's teeth, as we might do with a dog. We hadn't even discussed our options if Buzz persisted in refusing. And we still had so many misgivings. . . . Was there something else we hadn't tried yet, something better, healthier, more organic?

But suddenly Buzz was reaching for the pill.

"I'll take it," he said. "But I want it with tapioca, like Benny Schwartz gets."

He was looking at us with an unfamiliar expression.

Heaven help us. Was it trust?

A COUPLE DAYS AFTER Buzz took his first pill, I called up Blossom, his tutor, to tell her the news. I'd gotten in the habit of telling Blossom everything, as she had encouraged me to do. By then, I trusted her completely. Over the past few weeks, I'd told her all my fears and frustrations, and she'd been giving me the kind of support that I'd been craving for years.

After I mentioned the Concerta, however, there was a pause long enough to make me wonder if we'd been disconnected. Then she said: "I'm sorry to hear that. Because I can't tutor children who are drugged."

"What?"

"This has been my policy, for thirty years. I've always done it this way. I'm sorry you weren't aware."

Nope, I wasn't aware. How could I have been? She had never mentioned this, and it certainly wasn't in the contract we'd signed. . . .

I listened as patiently as I could, however, as Blossom suggested that Jack and I had decided too hastily, and wondered if I'd considered that Ritalin was actually *speed,* and that it turns kids into "zombies." Despite all I'd learned, I felt such a wave of new guilt that I actually started rethinking our hard decision. Maybe, I told Blossom, we'd suspend the meds for another month, until the end of the school year, and give her a chance to work her magic. Maybe I'd been exaggerating how bad things had gotten. Maybe Buzz hadn't really been crying out for help, as I'd imagined, that day with the knife. . . .

My frantic negotiations with Blossom spanned the next three days, including several e-mails and a couple of long phone calls. Our final conversation took place on a warm May evening, with chickadees twittering in our backyard pistache tree and jasmine scenting the air. Cradling the phone on my neck, I ducked into my writing shed to check my e-mail, half-listening as Blossom insisted on reading, in its entirety, a long letter from one of her grateful graduates "who has ADD but was never drugged."

There were two new messages, the first a one-liner from my psychiatrist sister, Jean, whom I'd briefed on the crisis. Jean is eight years older than I am, has two grown kids, and is much more matter-of-fact than I am about most things. She can wear a scarf or hat, for instance, without constantly tugging at it.

"Dump the fucking tutor!" her message read.

The second e-mail was from Blossom herself, forwarding a report from an Internet site on the by-then two-week-old campus shooting in Virginia by a deranged student named Cho Seung-Hui. "Are meds to blame for Cho's rampage?" asked the headline of a story that went on to quote Dr. Peter Breggin, speculating that Cho "might have been tipped over into violent madness weeks or months earlier by a drug like Prozac, Paxil, or Zoloft."

After reading these two e-mails, I typed and sent a reply to Blossom that ended up negating all my earlier attempts at conciliation. Let's just say it was the kind of message always better to save in your drafts file overnight.

Blossom's frosty reply arrived the following morning. "After taking everything into consideration," she wrote, "I have decided that it would be best for me to stop tutoring Buzz at this time."

I knew there was nothing I could do at that point, although it didn't keep me from second-guessing everything I'd said. By a lucky break, I had some work to do that evening in Santa Cruz, which gave me the chance to seek solace, afterward, from my novelist friend Sarah. Her son, now a college student, had ADD and a terrible temper, just like my Buzz. We headed to a bar, easily resuming the conversation that we'd been having for weeks about clinical distraction and meds.

"We used to call him Ballistic Boy, and sometimes Commando Demando," Sarah confided, as we huddled in front of the bar's fireplace, nursing margaritas. "The only time I ever felt close to him was when I'd go into his room and watch him sleeping. I'd stroke his head, and his face would be relaxed, and he'd seem like other kids."

I specifically needed to hear more about Commando Demando that night. I craved the honesty of other suffering mothers of "challenging" sons. Several months later, I'd come across additional consolation in a study by the psychologist Ilina Singh, who had interviewed a group of such mothers. She described them as anxious, desperate, and terrified, as they compared their experiences to being "trapped on a runaway train," or caught in a riptide. Asked to choose among several photographs for one that matched how they felt about themselves, several pointed to a picture of a *Tyrannosaurus rex*.

Sitting by that fire with Sarah, however, sixty miles from home, I finally started to relax, as we watched younger, miniskirted women check out the crowd, never dreaming of the fates to which their friskiness might lead. Sarah told me she had tried medication for

Commando Demando when he was Buzz's age, but probably sabotaged any hope of progress by stopping and starting and stopping again, out of guilt. A decade later, as she generously confided, she wished she had tried the drugs earlier and kept them up. She urged me to trust my instincts.

I told Sarah about Blossom, and together we cursed her perky name. I ignored my drink, tipsy with the delight of shared misery, as I steered the conversation once more back to Commando Demando. "Tell me again," I wheedled, "how he put his fist through the wall that time."

BUZZ TOOK HIS methylphenidate for less than a week before amazing things started happening. He put aside the Lakers jersey, gold chain, and sunglasses. Somewhere in his closet he discovered a neat white polo shirt, which became the keynote of his new school-day attire. Over the next couple of weeks, his meltdowns sharply declined. He stopped listening to rap. Two of his teachers called, unsolicited, to express their delight about his newfound focus. He smiled more often. Jack and I had feared he might develop facial tics, but instead, all the weird things that were going on before—the leaping eyebrows, shrugging shoulders, jerking lips—melted away.

I never imagined things could be this much better. Jack and I shook our heads at each other, mystified, as we watched Buzz knuckling down to his homework. He brushed aside my questions about how the pill made him feel, yet didn't once object to taking it, and once even said, "I think it makes me less impulsive." Meanwhile, I watched him happily taking in the world's new responses to his changed behavior. I was just about ready to write ads for Concerta.

I tried a pill or two from Buzz's supply, and—wow!—got a new perspective. I might still have been losing my keys, glasses, and pens, just the same as before, but I didn't *mind* half as much. Oh, right, I remembered: stimulants were originally prescribed as mood-elevators. In this case, they certainly helped persuade me that the ends justified the means.

I got my own prescription from Dr. Y. and took Concerta sporadically, just on days when I thought it might help. My threshold for boredom went up a few notches, helping me plow through some of the mind-numbing freelance editing work I'd taken on to cope with our skyrocketing therapy expenses. More importantly, I noticed that my threshold for Buzz was higher. His improving behavior, combined with my own goosed neurotransmitters, were dramatically reducing our clashes. He still tried to provoke me, but not as much, or as often, and I seemed to be handling it better. Researchers have confirmed these impressions, documenting a sharp decline in "negative" and controlling behavior by mothers after their ADD children started stimulants, and even improvement in the mothers' relationships with their husbands, and their sons' teachers.

When my father heard about our decision, he mailed me a picture he found on the Web: a billboard with a small boy's face and the motto: "Ritalin: So Much Easier Than Parenting." ("It's a joke [not a judgment!]" he scrawled.) Before the methylphenidate, I might have called him up and yelled at him, but this time I just tossed the note in the recycling box. And then I called Phil to apologize. We hadn't spoken for nearly a year, since the Hanukah party. I told him our saga, and all he said was, "You can't ever really understand something like this unless you go through it."

While certainly not all children respond as brilliantly as Buzz did, most do improve with medication. About 85 percent have a positive reaction to the first or second drug they try, although up to 15 percent suffer one or more of various side effects, including headaches, tics, weight loss, and increased blood pressure.

At most, Buzz had five nights of trouble falling asleep. I brought him mugs of warm milk with honey. His appetite waned for about a week, and then came roaring back. Over the summer, he went to a tennis camp and had a great time. He became really good at Ping-Pong. He made two new friends, one of whom invited him to his house. He was newly interested in books, moving quickly beyond Harry Potter to *The Kite Runner, Going After Cacciato,* and Jon

Stewart's *America*. He assembled a desk for his room all by himself, and once I even caught him helping Max with his Lego.

But I'm leaving the very best for last: after just that first week, he came up and hugged me and told me he loved me. And I realized that the last time he had done that was—a year ago? Two years? The fact is, I couldn't remember the last time.

It's enough to make you wonder—who are we, anyway? Where, inside our brains, is the "I" that's trying to be a better person? How much of what we've always thought of as willpower, character, even sheer morality, boils down to fluctuations in brain chemistry?

All good questions. But in that summer after our hard, hard year, I simply thought: who cares? My son was finally feeling better.

Mr. Hyde was gone, even though Mr. Intensely Annoying was still hanging around. That fight in our car in which he badgered me for coffee, and which set me on the path to write this book, took place four months after he had started the methylphenidate. Yet even while I suffered through it, I recognized how much worse it could have been before.

Reflecting on how close we came to disaster, I'd catch myself wishing we'd started the meds earlier. Like maybe right after that meeting with the Strattera-clock guy.

Jack and I still shared serious misgivings, however, including nagging worries about biased researchers and side effects perhaps yet to be documented. We were also both appalled by what seemed to be a growing national trend to use pills to boost kids' academic performance. To what extent, we asked ourselves, were we medicating Buzz to fit his square peg into the round hole of the flawed public school system?

I resolved to keep watching him carefully, and to keep up our regular meetings with his psychiatrist, Dr. Z., while I continued my research. If at any time the drugs' benefits waned, or side effects emerged, or a nonmedicinal alternative seemed promising, or the balance shifted away from short vs. dead, Buzz was going to go cold turkey.

The trick—always the hardest trick—would be to keep paying attention.

FOR SEVERAL DAYS after Blossom dumped us, I couldn't figure out how to tell Buzz. I didn't want him to link taking the pill with the loss of that fun, helpful relationship.

I ended up waiting for a moment when he was calm, and found it, once more, at our kitchen table, where he was eating a big plate of fusilli pasta, slathered with organic tomato sauce. He's usually in a good mood when he's eating.

"So tell me what you think about how it's going with your tutor," I began.

"She's great, but she's too expensive," he answered. "We could be spending the money on other things. Why don't *you* just do it?"

Oh my. That question again. Still, he wasn't asking me to home-school him. He was talking about maybe two hours a week. *Why didn't I just do it? We'd have stricter schedules, more enforceable rules, maybe the charts again. . . . I'd work harder, I'd—*

"I'll put out a shingle," I said. "What should I call myself? Leaf?"

"Roots," he said, without hesitation.

I swear I'm not making this up.

"You feel like roots," Buzz said.

So there we were. Roots and shoots. And I was newly determined to keep trying to push him toward the light—especially if he kept saying things like that.

CHAPTER 3

BIOLOGY

The Anatomy of Distraction

All children are essentially criminal.

DENIS DIDEROT

"*THERE'S* YOUR ADD!" SAYS DR. DANIEL AMEN.

The wiry, balding man with the kind brown eyes is pointing to a picture of a blue-and-purple-shaded, pockmarked blob. The image, which looks something like the little coral reefs you put in home aquariums, is a 3-D representation of my brain, captured by a nuclear imaging technology known as SPECT, for single photon emission computed tomography.

Earlier this morning, here in Dr. Amen's Newport Beach, California, office, a lab tech injected a formula containing a radioactive isotope into a vein in my right arm. The substance traced the flow of blood through my brain while I took a computerized concentration test. Then I lay on a table, while a multiheaded camera rotated around my skull, measuring gamma rays emitted by the isotope in my brain cells, all in the course of producing this image.

So *why* did I need this again?

The truth is that I've yearned for just this moment—with just this man, looking at just this sort of picture—ever since Buzz's grade school principal first suggested that he had attention deficit disorder.

She proceeded to recommend that I read up on Dr. Amen, the internationally best-selling author and clinician, who could look inside your brain and tell you exactly what was wrong, and why, and what to do. Four years later, still seduced by that vision of clarity, I've plunked down $2,100 for a scan and two-day clinical history, on top of a few hundred dollars more for the airfare and hotel.

I'm now five months into the year I'm devoting to my quest for clearer focus, having diligently stuck—*with only a few exceptions!*—to my plan of pushing other work aside to dedicate myself to reading, interviewing, and generally seeking whatever grains of truth might be found amid the fiercely competing viewpoints about clinical-grade distraction. My purpose in coming to Dr. Amen's clinic—a modest, one-story suite in a strip mall shared by two chiropractors, a neurofeedback clinician, and an acupuncturist—is to ascertain if "the Brain Doctor" can live up to his impressive advance billing, in which case I'll ask him also to scan Buzz.

I already know, from all that reading and interviewing, however, that this is one of those really big "ifs." While phenomenally successful, Dr. Amen is also one of the most controversial figures in the extraordinarily controversial field of psychiatry. He may be well ahead of his time; he may be saving lives—or he may, as many credible critics suggest, be pushing pseudoscience for a profit. Still, I'm shoving these questions aside, just for now, to focus on Dr. Amen as he taps his finger on the money shot: the part of the blue-and-purple blob where the hues pale to indicate what he says is lower than normal blood flow in my left inferior orbital prefrontal cortex.

"It's really quite mild . . . ," he hastens to assure me. But that's not why I'm grinning and nodding, peering over his shoulder. Seeing is believing, so they say. And just for this moment, I want nothing more than to believe in this quick 'n' easy explanation for the bedeviling brain glitch I share with my son.

YOU'D PROBABLY HAVE to have attention deficit disorder yourself, or be the parent of a child diagnosed with it, to share my interest in this picture. It's like looking at a close-up of Bigfoot or the Loch Ness Monster, or finding the smoking gun at the end of the rainbow. So many supposedly reputable experts—or, at least, experts prominently quoted in the media—insist that the disorder is a myth. Hysterical exaggeration. An avoidable product of vague cultural forces. "Biobabble." "The disease du jour." "Just being a boy." "A neat way to explain the complexities of turn-of-the-millennium life in America." The take-home message is it's all about a lot of spoiled kids and lazy parents.

Bolstering the champions of this view is the fact that more than a century of dogged research has yet to turn up an ADD smoking gun—or "biomarker." Dr. Amen's claims aside, the overwhelming mainstream scientific consensus to date is that there's no blood test or even brain scan offering undisputed membership in the club. Clinical distraction just isn't that kind of an either/or affair. It's more of a continuum—think blood pressure—with some potentially diagnosable people generally holding it together and others chronically overwhelmed. The cases are customarily diagnosed on the basis of a patient's (or that patient's parents') subjective responses to a checklist of behaviors—chiefly involving inattentiveness, hyperactivity, and poor impulse control—outlined in the ever-evolving mental health professionals' guidebook, the *Diagnostic and Statistical Manual of Mental Disorders,* or DSM. While most mortals are at least occasionally prone to some or all of these behaviors, the DSM says you're disordered if you've had six or more of them for at least six months, to a "maladaptive" extent. How is "maladaptive" measured? Again, it's subjective. But if this loose shoe fits, congratulations: you've got your diagnosis.

To be sure, the path is similar with most other illnesses we classify as mental, including depression, autism, and anxiety disorders. Yet in the case of ADD, researchers have pushed extra-hard to find that incontrovertible physiological evidence, which, not incidentally, would help justify physiological—i.e., pharmaceutical—treatment.

Many mainstream scientists dispute Dr. Amen's claim that he can diagnose ADD with a single brain scan, arguing that current technology simply isn't up to that extremely demanding task. Nonetheless, as even Amen's critics acknowledge, recent studies of large *groups* of brain scans link seriously scatterbrained behavior with differences in brain architecture and function.

Several brain structures are on average as much as 12 percent smaller—and also *less active*—than the norm in diagnosed children, these studies show. These parts include the frontal lobes, where Dr. Amen said he "saw" my ADD, the basal ganglia, the corpus callosum, and the cerebellum. The frontal lobes are famous as the seat of judgment, organization, and planning—the brain's so-called executive functions—while the other structures, in turn, play roles in initiating movement, regulating coordination and balance, and processing information. Researchers say their development in diagnosed children lags about three years behind that of other children, although it eventually catches up. Yet even in adulthood, in most cases, these brain structures remain relatively slothful, leading me to wonder: Do impaired frontal lobes explain why Buzz and I have made so many bad judgment calls? Are substandard basal ganglia to blame for my having to tell him six times to brush his teeth before he'll do it? Does a flawed corpus callosum suggest why I'm such a klutz, and might a pokey cerebellum hint at why we both so embarrassingly often need to ask people to repeat what they've just said?

Such conclusions are equally tempting and risky. Scientists still can't precisely explain how our brains manage such essential skills as attention, motivation, and self-control. Moreover, in some cases, at least, smaller brain structures may actually be more efficient, given that the brain develops by both growing neurons and "pruning" them. Even so, the brain-scan studies do seem to illustrate long-held ideas about serious distraction.

One of these ideas is that seriously distracted brains are "sleepy" brains, perpetually hungering for something to help wake them up. All brains, as a rule, love some degree of excitement, but these disabled, ADD brains *crave* it, indulging in risks, conflict, and/or rampant anxiety if they can't find more benign energizers. Looked at this way, when Buzz throws his scrambled eggs at Max, or bugs me for

$200 Kobe Bryant shoes after I've said no for the sixth time, it's really just his brain's way of sending out a frantic SOS, begging for a neuro-chemical hit.

What Buzz—and I—may well crave more than anything on such occasions is dopamine, a much-celebrated neurotransmitter under-lying attention and motivation. You might think of dopamine as the brain's elixir of excitement. It has the special role of alerting us to important novelty—the handsome dude, the snake in the grass, the check in the mail. It helps us move—forward to grasp, or backward, to flee. Too much can make us psychotic, while too little can liter-ally immobilize us, as with victims of Parkinson's disease. In recent years, scientists have gathered increasing evidence that ADD brains have a major problem with this vital chemical. They either make less of it, or use it less efficiently. Considering that dopamine levels tend to rise when you ingest caffeine, cocaine, or amphetamines, it starts to make sense that so many seriously distracted people end up turning to prescription or recreational stimulants to cope with their deficit.

Genetic researchers maintain that our hungry, sleepy brains are in most cases a family legacy. Disabling distraction, as they've found, is in fact more heritable than schizophrenia, and only somewhat less so than height. That's to say that only a minority of seriously scatter-brained people got that way because their pregnant mothers smoked or drank, or from falling on their heads or sniffing too many paint fumes.

As many as twenty gene variations, or alleles, may contribute to serious distraction by influencing the way the brain responds to neu-rotransmitters associated with attention. Here, too, the most inter-esting of these neurotransmitters is dopamine. In one key finding, scientists have discovered that a gene variation known as DRD4-7, and commonly found in people diagnosed with ADD, may somehow contribute to blunting the brain's response to dopamine, making people born with that allele unusually inclined to seek excitement and novelty.

I should stop to point out that novelty-seeking isn't always a bad thing—far from it. According to one popular theory, the DRD4-7 al lele and others like it helped our primitive hunter ancestors survive, since they needed to be extra vigilant about finding food while not becoming food themselves. When humans later settled down on farms, the restlessness became more of a liability, except when it came time to get out of Dodge—or Drubnin, as in the case of my great-grandfather Elias. The DRD4-7 pattern today is commonly found among migrants, particularly including descendants of the tribes that crossed over the Bering Straits to settle in North America. It thus seems plausible that Elias carried it along on his voyage to America, where he handed it down to my father, who fled his birthplace in Minneapolis after giving it to me, a future professional wanderer. And then, on a warm Southern Hemisphere summer night, most likely in Montevideo—after a day spent with Jack covering the Uruguayan presidential elections, followed by dinner at a cozy Italian restaurant—I bequeathed it to a microscopic Buzz.

FOR ALL THE scientific efforts to fathom clinical-grade distraction, there's still tremendous uncertainty about its origins, mechanics, and, above all, its optimum treatment. Dr. Amen flourishes in this void. He's a certainty-monger: the author, at last count, of twenty-two books, including the first book I read following Buzz's diagnosis, entitled, with characteristic optimism, *Healing ADD*. He lectures all over the world, while running four busy clinics, in California, Washington, and Virginia, where he calculates that he and his associates have scanned more than twenty-five thousand brains.

As I sit in his sunny office, still entranced by the image of that blue-and-purple blob, his cellphone rings—to the tune of the Scarecrow's lament in *The Wizard of Oz*: "If I Only Had a Brain"—but he graciously ignores it, launching into some welcome news.

"You've got a beautiful brain," he says, making it sound just a bit lascivious. "It's a brain that looks ten years younger than it is."

"I bet you say that to all the girls," I parry.

"No, really," he says, chivalrously assuring me that he only recently warned a *Vogue* reporter that she needed to cut down on the alcohol and coffee.

"I drink a *lot* of coffee," I retort. In fact, my lack of caffeine this morning, as required before the scan, may explain why I had to pull over my rental car on the way to Dr. Amen's office, after my cell-phone earpiece wire somehow got tangled around the steering wheel. As I'll soon find out, I've also botched that computerized attention test, which had seemed so simple at the time: my task was merely to mouse-click each time a letter that was not the letter X appeared on the screen.

"So what's going wrong?" I ask him.

"Your basal ganglia are working too hard," Dr. Amen tells me, tapping another part of the blob. "That's a sign of anxiety. And here's another hot spot, in your anterior cingulate, which suggests a tendency to over-focus."

It crosses my mind that Dr. Amen may have gleaned these insights from the questionnaire I filled out earlier, which asked, among other things, about my level of anxiety. But I leave that aside for the moment to bask in the narcissistic pleasure of watching him "read" my scan, like a palm or horoscope. I can feel my customary professional skepticism making way for a surge of transference—that warm, fuzzy feeling people get for psychotherapists—or, maybe, considering the circumstances, McTransference. What a confident voice he has! How earnestly he furrows his brow! No wonder Dr. Amen, a former altar boy, was voted "Most Friendly" at Vanguard University, the small Christian college where he got his BA. He's patient and engaged, full of smart insights, a skilled communicator with an edgy sense of humor. Yet how clearly am I really seeing him? I've got my notebook and tape recorder out, but the fact remains that I've come here at a time of desperation, in the thick of my struggles with Buzz, the tornado plowing through my world. Objectivity isn't my number one goal. I want answers; I want simplicity; I want "the Brain Doctor" to fix us.

And I yearn to believe that he knows how.

So pretty soon I'm back to Topic A, telling Dr. Amen how crazy Buzz is making me. He commiserates, telling me about all the parents he's seen who say they can't wait for their kid to turn eighteen.

Then he asks: "What's your worst worry?"

"That he'll end up in jail," I blurt out.

"Is that a *realistic* worry?" Dr. Amen asks.

Well, there he has a point. I worry more and, if I daresay, more imaginatively, than most other people I know. On the other hand, just two weeks before arriving here, I attended a lecture by the renowned attention deficit disorder expert Dr. Russell Barkley and after the first ten minutes felt an evidence-based desire to go home and put my head in the oven. Dr. Barkley has spent the past thirty years compiling statistics elaborating the disastrous life courses of so many people with ADD. He ran down the list, as I sat cowering on my aluminum chair. Teen pregnancies! Car wrecks! Suicide attempts! *Four times* as many sexual diseases. Many more encounters with police. Less satisfactory marriages. Fewer close friends. More impulse purchases. A higher frequency of vague medical complaints. Possibly more cancer. And most definitely much more immoral behavior, with an uncommon number of scatterbrains—and here, Dr. Barkley slowed down, to let it really sink in—growing up to be *cold-blooded predators.*

Dr. Barkley is a debonair Dr. Doom: a polished speaker with a tan face and neatly coiffed white beard. In a brief, post-lecture chat at the cheese-and-carrot table, where I pestered him until an aide whisked him away, he elaborated on an early influence on his research: a fraternal twin who was diagnosed with ADD as an adult after many bouts of homelessness, and who'd recently died in a car crash. Understandably passionate in his desire to prevent similar tragedies, he insists that children with serious attention issues should take meds throughout their lives, while extolling the special benefits of military service for young men with the disorder.

Military service. Buzz in a tank, at night, in Iraq. Back in Dr. Amen's office, I struggle to yank my thoughts away from scenes of car bombs, army hospitals, maybe even *military* jails. This subject is simply too painful, so I change it, darting back into reporter mode.

"Do you think *you* have ADD?" I ask.

"No, I have more of an anxious scan," he confides, his brow furrowing again. Hard work was a major value in his family, as he tells me. The son of a Lebanese grocery chain executive, he joined the army at eighteen, where he was trained as an X-ray technician, laying the framework for his lifelong preoccupation with looking at people's insides. He got his MD from the evangelical Christian Oral Roberts University and did his psychiatric residency at the Walter Reed Army Medical Center. He soon rebelled against his chosen profession, however, arguing that the aversion of most psychiatrists to using brain scans was "archaic, dated, and stupid."

In 1991, Dr. Amen began using SPECT scans to diagnose mental disorders: work, as he's written, that he believes has been "led by God." Indeed, desperate parents have flocked to this Newport Beach office as if it were a strip-mall Lourdes. One of these clients, a successful attorney, told me he sought out Dr. Amen after "at least a dozen" other therapists had failed to help his clinically distracted, oppositional, suicidal young daughter. Dr. Amen scanned the girl's brain, detected "very low temporal lobe activity," and, according to her father, vastly improved her behavior with a regimen including antiseizure medication and fish oil. "There's no question in my mind that he saved my daughter's life," the father told me.

At the end of my own two-day visit, which included the scan, a clinical workup, and two long conversations, Dr. Amen hands me a six-page report. He recommends that I continue taking Concerta and fish oil, and that I add ginkgo supplements to boost blood flow to the brain. He also wants me to read *Loving What Is,* by the self-help guru Byron Katie, to help learn how to deal with difficult thoughts (such as imagining Buzz in jail). I plan to follow up on all of them, I really do, but suspect what has already helped me the most was just to see that blue-and-purple blob, suggesting that maybe at least some of my many failures as a daughter, student, journalist, wife, and mom—the hotheadedness, the mistakes, even the messy behavior charts—aren't really my fault. This is the essence of Dr. Amen's magic: a surgical removal of shame.

"If he does nothing else," I enthuse to my mainstream-psychiatrist brother Jim, on the phone a few days later, "he helps so much just by the way he reframes things."

"Yes, it's kind of like phrenology," Jim coolly replies, referring to the broadly discredited nineteenth-century practice of analyzing personalities by examining bumps on the head.

"But he's helping people."

"Sure," my brother allows—"unless they'd be helped better somewhere else."

AS I'LL FIND, once I shake off enough of the McTransference to do more thorough reporting, Jim's retorts are actually an understated version of mainstream scientists' objections to Dr. Amen. The broad consensus is that brain scans, SPECT or otherwise, aren't yet up to diagnosing anything more subtle than a tumor. Part of the problem is that individual brains are just too variable. One person's "underperformance" may be normal for someone else. Furthermore, say the critics, Dr. Amen's claims have not been put to the test of rigorous, peer-reviewed studies.

"If somebody tells you, 'There's your ADD,' you should grab your purse and run," warns the widely respected neurobiologist James L. McGaugh, an expert in learning and memory at the University of California at Irvine. "This is really not like finding the break in a leg bone."

This view is so widely held that in 2005, a committee of the American Psychiatric Association issued a paper denouncing the use of SPECT as a clinical tool. "No published investigation has determined any brain abnormality is specific to a single psychiatric disorder," said the paper.

Dr. Amen and his many allies—among them Dr. Edward "Driven to Distraction" Hallowell, who has called him a "real pioneer"— suggest his foes may be jealous, resenting all that money he's earning with his clinics and books. What I suspect may be equally true is that the controversial brain scans call uncomfortable attention to how much of what psychiatry does—as helpful as it often is— amounts to guesswork. Dr. Amen may resemble the Wizard of Oz, a humbug behind a curtain, but many of his colleagues share the same stage, just without the cool special effects.

Returning from Newport Beach, I spend the next three weeks dithering over whether to bring Buzz in for a scan. I call twice to make appointments and then call back to cancel them. I seem to have lost my early faith.

It's not just the critics' complaints. I keep looking at Dr. Amen's six-page list of interventions, several of which involve instructions to buy his specially marketed supplements: his NeuroVite multiple vitamin, "developed specifically for our patient population," NeuroOmega fish oil (a brand he claims is the best on the market), and NeuroLink formula, containing GABA, 5HTP, taurine, and L-tyrosine.

While still caught up in McTransference, I buy two big white bottles of the NeuroLink formula, a six-week supply for $80. Dr. Amen said it would be good for Buzz, too, but before I give it to my son, I'm going to check it out. I e-mail the list of ingredients to Mc-Gaugh, the Irvine neurobiologist, who begins his reply by reminding me that the supplement industry remains almost entirely unregulated, freeing its merchants to make extravagant claims. As for NeuroLink's ingredients, he says: "I know of no evidence that would suggest that these substances would work as a brain supplement." My big white bottles end up in the back of my medicine cabinet, along with the detritus of other briefly hopeful splurges, such as the Mind Power Rx physician-formulated ginkgo biloba ("Supports Healthy Brain Function") and Dr. Perlmutter's NeuroActives Brain-Sustain formula ("for Enhancing Brain Function, Maintaining Memory, and Protecting the Brain").

I still want so much to believe in those scans. But not enough, in the end, to watch Buzz receive one of those radioactive isotope injections. The APA council's paper on SPECT specifically warns of the risks of such injections for children, who have greater sensitivity than adults to radiation, and possibly also greater risk for cancer. Dr. Amen, when I call to ask him about this, assures me the radioactive exposure from the average SPECT scan works out to about one-sixth of the exposure from the computed tomography scan (formerly known as a CAT scan) that doctors commonly order for orthopedic injuries, head trauma, and even abdominal pains. "You told me you were worried your son might end up in jail," he reminds me. "Isn't that more serious than a stomachache?"

Of course it is. Yet I keep thinking back to Jim's question of whether Buzz could be helped more somewhere else, i.e., without the injection. I don't want to make this decision by myself, so I ask Jack—a bit belatedly, I suppose—what he thinks.

"No way he gets scanned," he says.

Phew.

VEERING OFF THE brain-scan path sends me back to the grayer realm of conventional knowledge. I'm alone again in my writing shed, day after day, while the boys are in school, as I'm reading scientific journal articles and conducting telephone interviews with medical researchers. After just a couple weeks of this, I'm bored and restless, missing Dr. Amen's sparky aura of money and fame and insta-cures. Fortunately, this is when I meet Todd Rose.

I see him for the first time in a DVD shown at a lecture in San Francisco by the Utah psychologist Sam Goldstein, who diagnosed Rose with ADD back in the early 1980s and has been telling his remarkable comeback story ever since. On the video, Rose has the sweetest face—open and earnest, under his blond crew cut—*but what a troubled past!* His younger brothers cringe on camera, reminiscing about how he'd bully them. Rose tells of lying and loneliness, and how, growing up in his strict Mormon family, he used to pull off stunts including throwing a handful of stink bombs into the class of an art teacher he disliked. His father, on camera, says: "I always expected that he'd grow up to be a smart criminal."

At nineteen, after dropping out of high school with a .9 (that's no typo) grade point average, Rose got his teenaged girlfriend pregnant, and was working as a $4.50-an-hour stockboy. He was fulfilling all of the worst statistical predictions, until the birth of his baby inspired

him to start turning his life around. He returned to school and embarked on an academic career that has led to his current position as
a busy researcher and lecturer in Harvard University's Graduate
School of Education.

Before I even talk to him by phone, I'm imagining Rose—a happy
husband and father, engaged in an illustrious, altruistic career—as a
possible grown-up version of Buzz: a Buzz who didn't end up in jail,
after all; a Buzz who managed to find and follow his bliss, and who
might even be able to articulate why he couldn't walk past his brother,
just once, without punching him. Try as I have, I still can't get any
straight answers from Buzz himself, on this point or most others.
He's a resolutely closed book, and not just with me. I suspect the last
person he confided in was his tutor, Blossom, before she quit.

"Why do you think it's so irresistible to hit Max all the time?" I
ask, as I drive him somewhere, glancing over to see him staring at
the rearview mirror, fingers busy with his mouth.

"Buzz?"

He turns triumphantly, propping up a lopsided grin, and mum-
bles: "Harelip!"

I have so many stored-up questions I'm dying to ask Rose, but the
first thing he wants to talk about, once I track him down, by phone,
at Harvard, is how much he didn't want to do that DVD.

"I'm pretty competitive?" he says, his tone conveying bashfulness.
"I just wanted to be the best possible student. It's not like I wanted to
make a name for myself by saying, 'Hey, look, once I was a screwup?!
But now I'm not!'" But Goldstein persuaded him, he tells me, by reminding him of all the despair out there, and how much parents
need some example of success. Rose soon learned the truth of this.
After the rare occasions when he tells his own story in public, he
says, mothers tend to crowd around him in anxious clots of hope.

"Invariably they cry," he says, "and I'll cry, too. They'll say, 'You're
just like my Johnny!' and I'll say, 'I'm sorry!' I've learned from them
just how hard it was for my own mom. They feel so lonely, and so
worried they've somehow ruined their kids' lives."

Hey, that's me! That's me, too, Todd!

Rose, as it turns out, loves to talk, and he talks so fast it often seems to leave him breathless. He darts from subject to subject, cutting himself off in mid-sentence, cracking jokes and chuckling. I start laughing along, as it hits me that I speak his revved-up language. Scrunching the phone with my neck, I type as fast as I can, as he half-explains his half dozen different projects. *Have I got all this straight?* Rose works with a pioneering Harvard master's program called Mind, Brain, and Education. His main gig is to study a group of exceptionally talented astrophysicists diagnosed with dyslexia, which Rose thinks might help explain why they're so good at detecting black holes. He teaches neuroscience to grad students and also, over the summer, to inner-city adolescents in a special program at Brigham and Women's Hospital, in Boston. In the time left over, he chairs an institute that brings together academic faculty members from all over the country to learn about brain mechanics and education. He has also recently designed a neuroscience course for policy makers.

In the midst of all this, he graciously finds a total of three hours over the next two days to talk with me about the basics of ADD.

As soon as I can get a word in edgewise, I ask my most urgent question: why couldn't he stop hitting his brothers?

Rose laughs his tragedy-plus-time-equals-comedy laugh and says: "You know, I'll still walk down the road sometimes these days and see people eating at a sidewalk cafe or something, and think it would be really funny to scare them, like bang on the window. The difference today is that I don't do it. And that's a really big deal."

He likes to illustrate just how big a deal this is when he's lecturing to a class of undergraduates. Every once in a while, he tells me, he'll walk over to a student and kick him in the shin. "And I can see him initially want to jump up and fight me—but then there's this welling up of context, as he's thinking something like, *I'd better not. I might get in trouble. And my professor wouldn't do that if he didn't have a reason. . . .*"

This kind of thinking is known as "effortful control," Rose explains. "Most animals can't do it. But humans have an amazing ability to stop ourselves from acting on a gut response, to use past memories to shape our behavior." Alas, however, the ability is variable. Not all of us can pay attention to an impulse in time to judge whether kicking the professor, or throwing the scrambled egg, or eating the entire carton of ice cream, is really a good idea. While it takes the average person about 250 milliseconds to resist an impulse, Rose tells me, people with ADD consistently take about 50 milliseconds longer, which may not seem like much, but might make the difference in whether you can bite your tongue instead of telling off your boss, or even swerve your car to avoid a jaywalker. It's like playing that children's game of "red light, green light," and always losing.

And, oh, my, does this sound like Buzz. "PLEASE don't wipe your hands on the—!" *Too late.* "Move away from that stove!" *Oops.* "GET AWAY FROM YOUR BROTHER!" *Oh, no!*

Buzz has a passion for things that shock, explode, and perturb— Chinese firecrackers, stink bombs, those rubber bags you sit on that make noises like farts. Who caved in and helped him buy those things? Don't ask. But I'll give you a clue: it's the same person cleaning up the firecracker gunk on the patio.

When I drive with Buzz, he'll often urge me to honk at the car in front of us, just for fun. Our home life can be about as serene as an emergency room on New Year's Eve. I'll open a door and get squirted in the face with water from a spray bottle. "Now try the jet stream!" Buzz shouts, chasing me.

He bumps, hard, into Max, who emits that pitiful wail.

"I didn't mean to!" Buzz shouts.

"That 'I didn't mean to' is getting old!" I shout back.

"*You're* getting old!"

"Go to your room!"

"*You* go to your room!"

And I worry, again, about the risk that Buzz might ever mouth off like that to a highway cop in a bad mood.

Buzz's self-control glitch has been evident for several years, as I confide to Rose. Back when he was a toddler, Jack and I got into the habit of chanting, "Patience is a virtue," which he'd parrot back as, "Patience is a CHOOCHOO!" while laughing his little head off.

This was just a few years after Daniel Goleman published his landmark best seller *Emotional Intelligence*. The book particularly emphasized the key skill of self-restraint, describing the classic 1960s Stanford University experiment, which Goleman refers to as "the marshmallow test." The scientists offered a group of four-year-olds a challenge: if they could wait for just a few minutes while an adult ran an errand, they could have two marshmallows. If they couldn't wait, they would have just one.

"Which of these choices a child makes is a telling test," writes Goleman. "It offers a quick reading not just of character, but of the trajectory that child will probably take through life." Indeed, later studies found dramatic differences between the two groups. Those able to delay gratification grew into young adults with far superior academic skills—even higher SAT scores—who were more eager to learn, and more able to respond to reason and to concentrate, make plans, and follow through.

I waited until Buzz's fourth birthday to give him the test. Following the script, I handed him the marshmallow, left the room for three minutes, and returned to find—he'd licked it. I hid my distress about this for years before confiding it to my brother Jim, who with typical kindness tried to cheer me up by suggesting Buzz hadn't really broken the rule. "This could be a sign of real intelligence," he offered. "He discovered a loophole!"

But is this really something I can celebrate? There's a fine line between thinking outside the box and breaking rules in a way that shatters trust. And I knew even then that this shadow zone would be familiar ground for my son, as it has been, so often, for me. In my darkest moments, I mutter that the jury is still out on Buzz's moral character. On the other hand, I know that even with all the research I've done these past now six months, I haven't yet managed to answer his plea: I'm not even close to understanding him. So toward the end of February, I figure it's time to try a different path, one I'm told will give me the most detailed look inside Buzz's brain that can be had without an isotope injection.

WHEN I FIRST divulged my troubles with Buzz to Cliff Saron in Colorado, he suggested that I take my son in for diagnostic testing, a procedure that has grown in popularity among parents in recent years, with society's increasing awareness of the complex variety of childhood mental issues. It involves a battery of tests to screen for a range of potential cognitive and emotional problems, yielding detailed recommendations for treatment and, potentially, also accommodations at school. Many psychologists, especially in the most affluent and anxious U.S. coastal communities, now do nothing else.

Saron encouraged me to make an appointment with a pediatric neuropsychologist whom he knew in Berkeley, and whom I'll call Rachel Brown. "You'll get a map of his mind," he promised me. "Based on that information, you then do an infinite amount of variegated interventions. Five years later, he'll be a different kid."

I'm willing to sacrifice a lot for this goal, yet I'm shaken to learn that Brown charges $220 an hour—with an estimated twenty hours, at least, necessary to fully evaluate Buzz. My insurance won't pay for any of it, of course. "I take credit cards!" Brown cheerfully assures me. I say a quick prayer of thanks for my book advance, as fast as I'm using it up, and even as I feel a shiver of guilt. If any of these costly approaches pay off, they're still wildly beyond reach for all but a minority of Americans who either have the cash on hand or benefit from some pro bono arrangement. Most of the rest—always assuming they're lucky enough to have health insurance—have to make do with the kind of assembly-line care doled out by that guy with the Strattera clock. In contrast, here I am, resorting to what's starting to seem like a neurotrust: a seller's market targeted at upscale parents at their wits' ends. Resigned, I mark my calendar to take Buzz to Brown's office, an hour's drive away.

Our first appointment is scheduled for 9 A.M., and although Buzz promises the night before that he'll cooperate, 7:30 A.M. finds him well into his usual schoolday routine: head under the pillows, demanding five more minutes, and then another five. "Buzz," I say, gritting my teeth. "We've had this appointment for the past three months. If we don't get there on time, she is going to charge us anyway. Buzz . . . Buzz . . . BUZZ, it's $220 an hour!!"

I walk stiffly out of his room, pound my forehead with my fist, and glance at the kitchen clock. It's 7:45. Jack, bless his heart, goes in to try to reason with him.

I hear Buzz complaining that he shouldn't have to get up early on a Saturday morning. I tell myself I'll give it five more minutes, and finish making breakfast, while glancing at the newspaper. There's a story about how pine-bark beetles are migrating to new, warmer areas because of global warming and are now destroying trees that had been absorbing carbon dioxide, a process that in turn is speeding up global warming. But now I can hear Buzz getting up. I go in and stand over him after he finishes slowly pulling on his pants. *Shirt. Socks. Shoes. This is too. Much. Work.*

Eyes closed, he stumbles theatrically into the kitchen, scarfs down some waffles, and dons his white Dodgers hat, and we are on the road, miraculously, in time. Brown meets us in her waiting room, wearing a bright pink sweater and black tennis shoes, with her blond hair pulled back in a youthful ponytail. I like her right away; she seems so confident and upbeat. She directs most of her attention to Buzz, capturing his affection, too—I can see it—as she kneels to look him in the eye, with a big smile, to explain her plan for the day. "I like to figure out how people *think*," she tells him brightly. "Doesn't that sound *weird*? But everybody has a different thinking style. Your parents want to find out what *yours* is, because they want to make life as easy as possible for you."

Buzz is nervously picking at his fingernails, but at the end of Brown's introduction, he tilts his head back to favor her with a radiant smile. I sigh inwardly. *The magic of rapport!*

We head to the testing room. Walking behind her, Buzz, still smiling broadly, beckons me to lean down. "She creeps me out!" he whispers in my ear.

I bite my lip, intent on not giving him the satisfaction of laughing. Then I watch in growing wonder for the rest of the morning, as Buzz cheerfully does everything that Brown asks of him.

She begins by interviewing me, while Buzz waits outside her office. She asks me several questions, following up on my answers on the questionnaires I've filled out at home, earning my immediate gratitude by not even seeming to notice that I'd (*or could it have been someone else?*) scrawled a grocery list on the back of one of them. Then she talks to Buzz, who also has to answer several pages of written questions.

For the rest of the time, a full eight hours over two days, Brown gives Buzz a series of cognitive and emotional tests, measuring his powers of attention, IQ, vocabulary, and reasoning ability. In one test, Buzz must assemble colored blocks according to different patterns she shows him. In another, she reads a list of words he must try to repeat back, first right away and then after thirty minutes.

Buzz took a series of similar tests several years ago, when he enrolled in that behavior-modification course at the University of California in San Francisco. But Brown's battery is much more extensive. "We are not just diagnosing a disorder," she has told me. "We are understanding a person."

For some of the tests, I stand or sit behind Buzz, peering over his shoulder, which Brown says she'll allow on the condition that I can restrain myself from butting in. This, as I soon find, is all but impossible. I want to take the tests for him, to help him do well. I watch intently, as Buzz—*such a good boy!*—answers a series of questions designed to test his reasoning powers. He's sniffing occasionally, as if he has a cold, which he doesn't. *Maybe it's a facial tic. Is this too much pressure?*

"What's the connection between sand and glass?" Brown is asking.

"Glass is made of sand," Buzz answers promptly.

"Cars and airplanes?"

"They're means of transportation."

(*That's my son!*)

"Mass and energy?"

"Both are different forms of the same thing." (*He's an Einstein!*)

But then Buzz has to choose among a group of pictures to find the ones that have something in common, and he's not getting the trick. The trick is to pick the things that are salty. Why can't he figure it out? *A pretzel, a pickle, and the ocean!* I want to scream, until I force myself to look out the window. For the first time this morning, I hear the sound of birds in the trees along the busy street outside. *Are these trees also being chewed away by beetles?* I turn my eyes back to the room.

"Why do we put license plates on cars?" Brown is asking.

"So the government can get money."

"Why do we have appellate courts?"

"To make sure things are fair, like if the first judge didn't understand something, or was prejudiced."

I need to slam on my own mental brakes to check an urge to rush over to embrace him. Maybe I've been all wrong about Buzz. Maybe he's blooming right before my eyes. Whispering an excuse, I run out to the grocery store down the block to buy him an eclair.

TWO WEEKS LATER, on a Monday when Jack is off work, he and I drive back to Berkeley, this time without Buzz, to meet with Rachel Brown. She hands us a ten-page typed report that includes Buzz's test scores and her interpretations.

As Brown starts talking, Jack and I glance at the first page and share a hearty chuckle at her opening description of Buzz as "amiable." Still, her positive impression of our challenging boy is encouraging, and there's even more to come. "Academically, he's awesome," Brown is saying. "He has incredible skills in reading and math, and amazing verbal ability." I stare at her report as she reads. It's true! In a test of math reasoning, he scores in the 94th percentile. In "numerical operations," whatever that is, but it sure sounds worthwhile, he's in the 99th. Yay, team!

But now she moves on to Buzz's handicaps, some of which appear to be quite serious. In fact, her report applies variations of the word "struggling" to Buzz a full seventeen times, describing him as so "anxious, sad, and lonely" that we should consider medication, beyond the methylphenidate, to treat it. This sets off immediate alarms. Not another medication quagmire! Plus I simply don't buy this analysis; Buzz, to me, seems so much more angry than sad. I murmur some protests, as Brown insists his rebel attitude is sheer facade, a tough-guy pretense of being in control, when, as she goes on to show us, he so clearly isn't.

She has noticed Buzz's restlessness during the test-taking—how he fidgets in his seat, tunes out when he's even slightly bored, and breaks rules, repeatedly trying to keep answering questions after the timer rings. Moreover, the speed at which Buzz processes information turns out to be just average, in the 50th percentile. For someone who scored average in other areas, this might not be a problem. But Buzz 's verbal skills can make it seem as if it's all coming easily to him, leading teachers, friends, and, yep, even parents, to expect more than he can deliver. A similar gap shows up when it comes to Buzz's "working memory," where he scores in the 61st percentile.

Working memory involves holding at least two things in your mind—things as basic as where you're going and how to get there. It's a vitally important skill that we use all the time and is also a common problem for people with attention issues. Ageing can sap working memory, but usually nowhere near the extent that clinically distracted people confront. One theory chalks this up, again, to a problem with dopamine, that precious molecule that helps kick your brain into action.

As Brown talks about the problems that poor working memory can cause, particularly in the classroom, I suddenly remember watching Buzz, at age three, opening the refrigerator door in our Rio de Janeiro apartment and asking himself, "What am I looking for?" I'd thought it was so cute and precocious at the time. And then I remember all the times I've been so mad at him for not being able to follow the most simple compound instructions, such as "Go brush your teeth and wash your face and get to bed!" And how he's had a hard time managing such rudimentary tasks as just bringing his homework home, and gets so touchy when I nag him about it.

"Most kids would naturally get punished for these kinds of mis-takes," Todd Rose will tell me later. (Rose says his own working memory score is in the *bottom 2nd percentile*.) "But when you punish for things that aren't in a child's control, it creates a really bad spiral. These kids are at a tremendous disadvantage, because as smart as some of them seem, they're going to fail at these simple things. They get told to try harder, and then they fail again. Sometimes they stop trying altogether, because trying is all they have left: if they try as hard as they can and still fail, they've lost it all."

The more we learn from Brown, the more it seems that Buzz's behavior has been less *dis*obedience than *mis*obedience. The clincher is when she describes one simple test that has revealed his excep-tionally weak impulse control. Buzz was told to tap his finger on the desk every time he heard a beep, but to stop tapping when he heard another tone. He missed the cue so many times that he scored in the 16th percentile for this task. "Compare this to sitting in a classroom where you can talk, but are expected to stop when you see the teacher stand up and walk to the blackboard," Brown explains. "All the other kids will attend to that cue, but Buzz will keep talking, with the result that his name gets called and he gets scolded, time after time after time."

Might Brown actually be on to something when she says Buzz is so sad? I could see how hard he was trying to cooperate with her, and still so often screwing up. Particularly poignant was his effort to copy a diagram she had shown him briefly, in which he'd entirely failed to capture the largest features—a big rectangle and triangle—even though he diligently reproduced many of the smaller details. It hit me then that he actually sees the world differently than I do—and that he's literally not getting the big picture.

Jack and I are finally starting to understand one big picture our-selves: that saying that Buzz "has ADD" comes nowhere near to telling his story, or helping us figure out how to help him. Our new informa-tion offers this more refined perspective: he's a gifted kid who is si-multaneously seriously handicapped by impulsivity, a weak working memory, and poor organizational skills. It feels like a breakthrough.

And now Brown is moving on to give us several practical suggestions. She thinks Buzz should stay on the stimulants, which she believes help give him a little more time to exert self-control. But we can also show Buzz's teachers her report to help them understand him better and, she hopes, to be less frustrated and judgmental about this seemingly bright boy who keeps missing the boat. We can ask for accommodations, including that Buzz be seated away from potential distractions such as talkative kids or open windows, and that his teachers monitor him more closely to make sure he understands what they're saying. We can get him yet another after-school tutor and sign him up for a workshop in organizational skills ($195 for three hours), which Brown says is given each summer by an "awesome" educational specialist.

Driving back under cold, gray skies, across the San Rafael Bridge, Jack and I mull over Brown's findings. We eventually agree that we're going to follow every one of her suggestions except for looking into further meds, at least for now. Our conversation keeps returning to the drama of those two geometric pictures, symbolizing the poignant doggedness with which Buzz appears to have been going about things all wrong.

"It kind of gives you more sympathy for him, doesn't it?" I venture.

"It's like he really just doesn't get it," Jack says. "Like when he says people are being mean to him, and he doesn't realize he's been a jerk. Maybe he doesn't even really remember what he has said or done. He has blind spots."

"When I look at him now when he's pestering me, I'll just picture a brain scan with underactive frontal lobes," I joke.

So this is the gist of my platinum-plated new frame of reference: the product of more than $6,000 in bills, so far, for my visit to Dr. Amen and for Buzz's diagnostic testing. But carping aside, I do finally feel as if I'm on more solid ground. Both Jack and I are now convinced there's really something to this ADD business, as vague as the label remains, and that we're dealing with basic biology, not Buzz's moral character or all the ways we've blown it as parents. And I'm more convinced than ever that Buzz was inspired to send me on this quest to understand him.

Todd Rose tells me that what can make the most difference when you're saddled with disabling distraction is the degree to which you're willing to be aware of and manage your eccentric makeup. I've heard variations on this theme before. Dr. Edward Hallowell eloquently calls the disorder "the gift that's hard to unwrap." The psychologist Lara Honos-Webb, author of *The Gift of ADHD,* goes so far as to argue that telling a restless child that he has attention deficit/hyperactivity disorder is like telling a woman she has "penis deficit/hypermammary disorder."

"Just as women's anatomical differences allow them to birth and feed babies—something men are not equipped to do," says Honos-Webb, "children with ADHD have abilities that other children don't have."

I know I've already seen glimpses of the gifts Buzz may one day unwrap. It's like the way my dad used to joke around when I was growing up. He'd open his mouth and point down his throat, saying, "Somewhere in there is a thin man, trying to get out! Listen, you can hear him!"—and he'd imitate the thin man's voice, calling: "Help! Help!"

All children may well be "essentially criminal," as Diderot said. And more so for children born unusually impulsive and distracted. Still, somewhere inside my son, I'm learning to trust, there's a *good* man, just trying to get out.

CHAPTER 4

RELATIONSHIPS

The Cookie of Peace

*The craving for appreciation is the
deepest principle in human nature.*

WILLIAM JAMES

IT'S 6:15 A.M. ON A MONDAY IN MARCH, AND I'M MIXING A DASH
of vanilla into the eggs for French toast. Sunlight spills through
the kitchen window, illuminating all the scratches and stains and
permanent marker scrawls on our breakfast table.

Buzz, on his own, has enrolled in a seventh-grade, pre-period
Spanish class—a welcome sign of academic motivation that I pay for
with the daily Herculean task of getting him out the door and en
route to his bus by 7 A.M. I predict that our school district will finally
get around to adjusting its schedules to conform with documented
adolescent diurnal rhythms on the day Buzz graduates high school.

I squeeze oranges and distribute each family member's vitamins,
fish oil, and meds among four saucers. Grind coffee beans, fetch
newspapers, and head to Buzz's room for the first wakeup call.

"Time to get up, honey!"

He grunts.

*Where's Jack? Still in bed? Oh, right, he worked the late shift last
night. It wouldn't be fair to expect him to be up by now.* Back in the
kitchen, the PBS radio station is announcing the start of another

fund drive. *A better person would be dialing that 1-800-number right now, checkbook in hand.* Instead, I'm frying some of those little chicken sausages Buzz likes, which I made a special trip to buy. *Protein in the morning is key. . . . But shouldn't he be making his own breakfast by now?*

Returning to Buzz's room, I switch on the light. "Let's go, sweetie!" No response.

"Buzz, you'll be late. Get up right now!" I shake his shoulder. Eyes still closed, he stretches his arms luxuriously. *He's toying with me. . . .*

I hear, from under the covers, a fart.

Arteries contracting, I head back to the kitchen and glance at the *New York Times* front page—more street bombings in Iraq—before I hear the bathroom door slam. He's up!

Ten minutes later, however, the shower is still running. I glance at the clock and knock on the bathroom door. "Buzz, there's no *time*. You need to eat breakfast and get dressed." No answer.

Another three minutes pass. I pound my fist on the bathroom door, to the rhythm of my thumping heart.

"BUZZ!!!!"

But then, four minutes to show time, and—a miracle! He's at the table, water dripping from his crew cut. *Why isn't he eating?*

"Finish your *breakfast*," I say.

He finally catches my eye.

"Say you appreciate me."

"*What?*"

"Say you appreciate all my hard work."

"Buzz, are you *kidding*?"

It's easy, in retrospect, to imagine what a better, smarter mother would have done in my place. I can just see her, in her apron, walking over and tousling his hair. *Sure, I appreciate you!* she'd say. End of story. Why can't I be that smarter mother? Why can't I say that simple thing? I'll tell you why: I'm *steamed* not only from the last half hour of noodging him awake, but from the last *four years* of conflict, frustration, disrespect, disobedience, towels on the floor, dishes in the sink, accumulating bills, deferred ambition, declining health, global warming . . .

Buzz has his arms crossed. He's saying something. *Huh?*

"I said I'm not doing anything more until you say you appreciate me."

"*Damn* you!"

Who just said that? Who actually said that to her own son? Who just lunged at him, grabbing his arm?

Now Buzz is crying. "I'm not going to school!" he says.

And *this* is when Jack walks into the kitchen.

He hasn't seen any of the sausage-buying and frying and French toast making, or the gentle, first waking-uppings. He sees only the frothing mom and weeping, victimized child. He looks at me not quite accusingly, but more searchingly than I think is fair.

"She wouldn't say she appreciated me! She swore and hit me!" Buzz shouts.

"Did NOT hit him!"

By this time, the noise has awoken Max, who sticks his head out of his room, sizes up the situation, and runs for his violin. He knows I usually love it when he plays. So now Buzz and I resume our shouting match over the tinny strains of the Gavotte from *Mignon*.

"Just get to school!"

"Fuck you!"

This time, I don't respond. This, after all, is what the parenting gurus teach: you don't feed the monster of abominable behavior with attention. Besides, I'm stricken by my *own* abominable behavior. Also besides, he's heading toward the door and I need him to keep going—even though there's no way by now that he's going to catch the bus in time for Spanish. Stalking to my bedroom, I close my eyes, catch my breath, and wonder, once again, what just happened.

Maybe Buzz really wasn't toying with me. Maybe he was simply lost in his own world, unaware of the water-torture impact of his behavior. And maybe I was unfairly aiming at him some of the outrage I should have reserved for the boneheaded school district, or the awful Iraq War. . . .

I race through the house, looking for my keys. They're not in the chipped ceramic bowl on the counter near the door, the new place

I'm trying to teach myself to leave them. They're not in my purse, or on my desk, or in my jacket pocket—*oh, thank God! They're under the bag of oranges. . . . How'd they get there? No time to wonder—*

Driving to the bus stop, I see Buzz standing alone. *His backpack looks too heavy for him; why haven't I noticed that before?* We smile at each other as he climbs into the car. In the past ten minutes, we've morphed into completely different people: smaller, quieter, better.

There's silence for most of the ten-minute drive, after which I venture: "Buzz, it's as if I'd made you horse manure for breakfast and stuck your nose in it and said, 'Why don't you appreciate it?'"

"It's not the same thing," he says, grinning.

"I appreciate you *now*," I say, and kiss his head before he hops out of the car and then turns, just for an instant, to wave good-bye.

I DRIVE HOME SLOWLY, zap some coffee in the microwave, and carry it out to my writing shed, turning over the events of the last hour in my mind.

Despite our continuing fireworks, Buzz and I have generally been working harder to get along, and I think we've made some progress. While we still fight—a lot—it's less often and less hurtful. Some of this may be owed to the methylphenidate, which we've now both been taking for almost a year. But I strongly suspect that what's helping just as much is the new way I've started to pay attention—slowing down, trying harder to tune in, and questioning my assumptions. Often, when Buzz starts to exasperate me, or when I'm tempted to respond in kind to his UpYours@hotmail.com take on the world, I work to keep in mind what I've learned from my Harvard ADD wilderness guide, Todd Rose, and Rachel Brown, the neuropsychologist— that Buzz is a kid who got needy for a reason, that he's been told "No!" and "Wrong!" and "Bad!" too many times, and that he just might be trying as hard as he can to do his best.

This new perspective has also made me think a lot harder about the second part of Buzz's diagnosis, at age nine, when researchers at the University of California at San Francisco tagged him not only with attention deficit disorder, but also with oppositional defiant disorder, ODD.

ODD first appeared in the *Diagnostic and Statistical Manual* in 1980, the same year that ADD made its debut. It's an equally murky prism, diagnosed in a similarly subjective way, its hallmarks including: losing one's temper, arguing with adults, refusing to follow rules, deliberately annoying people, and blaming others for one's own mistakes. Strikingly, as many as 65 percent of children diagnosed with ADD also qualify for ODD, which psychologists say subsequently risks developing into the next higher level of antisocial behavior: conduct disorder, characterized by behaviors such as bullying, torturing animals, arson, breaking into cars, and running away from home.

Such diagnoses reflect a modern trend to medicalize rather than moralize. Yet this remains still a minority point of view. In most of the world, kids who'd qualify for ODD or conduct disorder are still seen as budding or blooming juvenile delinquents, more deserving of a locked cell than a doctor's care. Parents who spare the rod will only make them worse, according to this popular view.

What proponents of each of these views often fail to appreciate, however, is a reasonable sense of context. Opposition and defiance are reactions, after all. The child is defying and opposing *some*body. Early on, that somebody is most often his mother, if only because she's closest at hand. On the other hand, she may also be fanning the flames.

Is it maternal sacrilege to point this out? We moms, after all, have so frequently and often so unfairly been charged with ruining our children. In the 1950s, the mostly male medical leadership decreed that cold, "refrigerator mothers" made children autistic, while "schizophrenogenic mothers" put voices in their heads. The widely revered Bruno Bettelheim went so far as to compare mothers of autistic children to Nazi concentration camp guards.

These unlucky and cruelly censured mothers must have felt as if they'd been mugged after being struck by lightning. It's easy to imagine their relief when new research sent the pendulum flying toward our current widespread belief that genes are the chief determinants of our children's destinies. The psychologist Judith Rich Harris took this argument to the extreme in her celebrated 1998 book, *The Nurture Assumption,* suggesting that genes outweigh the influence of almost anything parents might do, beyond criminal neglect or abuse. And what a reprieve that was! Or at least it was until newer research findings pushed that pendulum back yet again, offering persuasive evidence that parents' day-to-day behavior really does matter quite a lot.

Consider, for instance, McGill University scientist Michael Meany's pioneering discovery, in 2004, that the extent to which a mother rat licks and grooms her babies can determine whether certain genes in the pups' brains are turned on or off. As adults, the better-nurtured rats release less of the stress hormone cortisol when startled and tend to be generally less fearful. Testing a related hypothesis in humans, Michael Posner, at the University of Oregon, has shown that unskillful parenting—for instance, being dictatorial or cold—increases the odds that children born with the DRD4-7 allele, the gene pattern linked to risk-taking, will develop an attention disorder.

Meany's and Posner's findings fit in with a new wave of science known as epigenetics, informed by the understanding that influences from your environment—including your parents' behavior—influence the way your genetic blueprint unfolds. Nurture really can trump nature. And since women—despite all our supposed advances—still do the lion's share of child-rearing, we're on the hot seat for blame when things go wrong.

Right! So now we can get back to mom-bashing, okay? Well, not so fast. Because mothers don't live in a vacuum, either. As research reveals, our children are doing a number on us even as we do our number on them.

It was once assumed, for instance, that intrusive, controlling mothers were making their kids hyperactive. Then scientists found that when these kids took stimulants, improving their behavior, the moms nagged less. The moms' nagging, in other words, was a reaction to and not a cause of the children's behavior. In one imaginative project—a "child swap" made-to-order for reality TV—researchers

went so far as to temporarily switch mothers of children with conduct disorder (that serious escalation of oppositional defiant disorder)
with mothers of "normal" kids. In no time, the "normal" mothers
were pestering and criticizing, while the original naggers had chilled.

Thus, an innately challenging child can easily wear down the average parent, and in particular the scatterbrained parent. The child's
extraordinary resistance leads that parent either to back off or resort
to harsh punishment, making the child even more angry and aggressive. And so on, and so on, until everything falls apart—much like it
did for us during Buzz's eleventh year.

WHILE METHYLPHENIDATE HELPED break our downward spiral
during that terrible time, Jack and I never believed it would solve all
our problems. Nor did Buzz's psychiatrist. "The medication is just
one part of the plan," Dr. Z. told us, as he handed over the first prescription. "There are two other parts that are just as important. The
first is that Jack is going to have to get more involved. Buzz needs
his dad."

At this, I clasped my hands to check my urge to applaud. I'd been
nagging and sulking for years over this very point. While Jack hadn't
been completely out of the loop, he was so often absent, off working by day, or so exhausted, on evenings and weekends, that all he
wanted once he got home was to sneak off with his newspaper. As
sorry as I was to see him that tired, I thoroughly enjoyed Dr. Z.'s scold-
ing, until he added: "And *both* of you should get some professional
help with your parenting."

Hey, unfair! I thought, as he handed me a card with the name of
a parenting coach. I've already read enough parenting books to paper
over a small city. What good advice had I possibly not heard? Peeved,
I put Dr. Z.'s suggestion out of my mind for the next several months,
preferring to focus on that part about how Jack should change.

Focusing on how Jack should change has in fact kept me busy
nearly ever since we first met, on a muggy morning in 1982, at a government press office in Managua, Nicaragua. I was on one of those

working vacations, while Jack, then still a career freelancer, had won
a grant to report on the U.S.-backed revolt against the leftist Sandinista government. Smitten by his gray-green eyes, muscular arms, and
habit of making Yiddish wisecracks about the pompous Sandinista
officials, I'd maneuver to sit by his side at the open-air cafe under
palm trees, next to the Intercontinental Hotel, where reporters traded
stories while sipping iced cacao drinks.

Eleven years my elder, and without a steady job, Jack was living,
between reporting trips, in the back room of a shared Berkeley apartment, which we came to call "the crawl space." Until my parents got
to know him, they kept asking whatever happened to that nice law
student I used to date. Over the next eight years, we courted, fought,
and reconciled, while I anguished over how I could possibly share my
life with someone who seemed so averse to steady work and material
comfort—someone so alluringly and worryingly different from my
father. I kept it up until my exasperated shrink, Dr. Y., broke his professional silence to say, "Jack is good for you. You just have to let Jack
be Jack."

So I went ahead and married him, on a sunny afternoon in Men-
docino, California, and after twenty years am still grateful for Dr. Y.'s
advice, even as I only rarely manage to follow it.

Many clinically distracted people end up picking exactly the wrong
kind of spouse, writes Dr. Edward Hallowell. We think we need someone much more disciplined than we are, so we go to the extreme and
find "a caricature of a bad fifth-grade schoolteacher . . . controlling,
demeaning, belittling, and very well-organized." That's one mistake,
at least, I haven't made. Bless Jack's heart, he seems to love me as I
am. Our temperaments are also complementary. Jack's never in a
rush, unless he's late for a movie, and will schmooze with the pizza
delivery guy, while I'm checking my watch. I admired and cherished
his equanimity right up to the time I started to fret that he should
be much less cool and collected about Buzz.

No amount of my fretting ever moved him, however. It took Dr.
Z.'s masculine timbre to get the message through, or maybe it was
the sight of that prescription—concrete evidence of the depth of our

crisis. All I know is that from that day on, Jack paid more and better attention both to Buzz and to Max. He started taking the kids out to play basketball or to matinees on Sundays, giving me a couple extra hours to work. He'd say things like "Listen to your mother," after hearing me tell Buzz for the fourth time to pick up his wet towel from the floor. He began hanging out in the kitchen more and even waking up earlier to roust Buzz from his bed, something he told me was "taking a bullet for you"—until I asked how the hell it ever got to be *my* bullet.

But after that, I bit my tongue. Somehow we'd stumbled out of our angry rut and into what scientists call a positive feedback loop. As Jack made more of an effort with Buzz, I praised him effusively, which energized him to do even more. I stopped complaining quite so much and started finding ways to show him how grateful I was for all his efforts, explicitly linking my cooking of a brisket with his getting the kids out of the house. Retro? You bet! Effective? Damn straight!

Buzz was right, once again, to make his stand about appreciation. It may be the world's best motivator. But like most good things, it takes special attention. You have to be able to slow down enough to switch your focus away from all the ways things could be better, to how good they already are. Once I started doing this with Jack, it became downright embarrassing to notice all the things I might have appreciated earlier. Like how often he was doing the dishes—singing "Cinderfeller, Cinderfeller!"—and how he patiently talked sports and pointed out interesting things in the newspaper to Buzz and practiced the violin with Max. And how faithfully he had been calling me from work each day, especially during those difficult, long after-school afternoons. "Everybody still alive?" he'd ask, or, on better days, "What are you wearing?"

I gradually realized that "letting Jack be Jack" meant keeping my eyes fixed on his best side, the only side I saw when I first fell in love. The more I've been able to do that, the more that best side has emerged, and the happier all of us have been. Which is not to say there haven't also been many weekend mornings when the kids have been up pestering and fighting and I've been doing laundry, while he's been sleeping late, like a prince, and I've stalked into the bedroom, growling, "So, how much longer are you going to just LIE THERE?"

IT'S NOW A YEAR AFTER that embarrassing session with Dr. Z., and I'm heaving sheets and towels into the drier, on another of those endless after-school afternoons. *For this I went to Stanford?* I've just sent both of the boys to their rooms, after Buzz stabbed Max with a pen, and Max scratched Buzz's face, leaving a deep red claw mark, forensic evidence that his mother forgot to trim his fingernails.

Dr. Z. has called this our "cabin fever" problem. "You just have to get through this time," he told me. "Pretty soon, they'll both have other activities to keep them busy."

Perhaps I'm oversensitive to all this aggression, but I come by it honestly. During my own childhood, my two lively older brothers—today both not only my beloved friends, but exemplary family men and respected members of the medical establishment—tortured me endlessly, teasing me about my weight, throwing spitballs in my food, barging into my bedroom while I was dressing, and at one point fracturing my sternum (by stepping on it). While I recognize the trap of responding to the past in the present, it makes me no less resolute to prevent serious injuries on my watch.

I used to think my family was unusual in this respect, but I've come to doubt that. Among the things parents know today that no one seemed aware of—or ready to admit—when I was growing up is the extraordinary prevalence of sibling violence. Throughout America, brotherly and sisterly mayhem is much more common than that between husbands and wives or parents and children. A large study in 2005 found that more than one-third of siblings interviewed said they'd been "hit or attacked" by a brother or sister within the past twelve months, with nearly half of the victims having been assaulted repeatedly, leaving bruises, cuts, chipped teeth, and broken bones.

It's all about survival of the fittest, of course. Siblings are locked in competition for limited supplies of parental attention and resources. Who's getting more food? Or praise? If the house caught on fire, who'd be carried out first? In this way, the extra attention Buzz has gotten from being the "problem child" weighs on his brotherly bond with Max. In his efforts to even things out, Max publicly plays up his good-guy attributes while privately goading Buzz to misbehave. He has mastered the art of the subtle tease that sends Buzz crashing across the room in rage.

"Max, you're my angel," I once cooed to my younger son, in an unguarded moment when we were alone.

"And Buzz is your devil!" he immediately responded.

Max has been like this for as long as I can remember. While Buzz, as an infant, had kept me up all night, night after night, his little brother slept soundly for long stretches right away, waking in the morning light with a sweet, questioning look, as if to say, *Hey, I don't want to be a bother, but if you're not otherwise occupied, might breakfast be available anytime soon?*

Today, as Buzz remains moodily reticent, Max delivers charming, detailed bulletins on the goings-on at school and writes me memorable mash notes, like, "Mommy is sweet as a donut!" Instead of further splintering my focus, Max has adapted. Rather than lose things, he finds things that I lose. He calls from school to leave messages like "Mommy, just a reminder, I'm taking the bus home today. Bus, bus, bus, bus, bus!"

Piglets are born with a special set of temporary "needle teeth" to fight for the frontal teats with the most nutritious milk. Max deploys his charm, energetic curiosity, and a strategic knack that Gen. George S. Patton might have envied in his struggle for scraps of my attention.

"*Sacre bleu!!*" he'll shout, apropos of nothing.

"Mom, I think I know why there's a tear in the ozone layer. It's because of all the balloons that get lost, right?"

"Could a lion eat an elephant?"

"It takes 206 licks to get to the end of a Tootsie Pop, and they said the world would never know!"

Is it any wonder Buzz is—let's be generous—ambivalent about Max's existence?

Already, in an effort to reduce the risk of nocturnal assaults, I've moved Buzz out of the bedroom he'd shared with Max and into what we'd previously called "the family room." As soon as Buzz hit the minimum weight, we also let him sit in the front seat of the car, to prevent slugfests while I'm driving. But then comes a moment after I reprimand Max for some reason, and notice how beautifully Buzz starts to behave. The effect is instantaneous—more potent than any pill. I try it again. "Max, you are being *much too noisy!*" I say, and watch, from the corner of my eye, as Buzz's face becomes composed, serene, the jitters released from his body.

It feels at first like shameful manipulation, but, while trying not to overdo it—and while taking pains to follow all the good advice I've read about giving "normal" siblings opportunities to vent their complaints—I reprimand Max a bit more often in Buzz's presence. I do so only when he really deserves it, *of course.* And yet the more I tune in, the more I notice ways that he really so often does deserve it, like those whispered little singsong insults that he thinks only Buzz can hear.

Then one night it hits me how annoyingly Buzz hovers and interrupts, pinches and pokes, when I read to Max before he goes to sleep. The reading is nominally open to both boys, but it takes place on what is now Max's turf, in the room they used to share.

Buzz is twelve. Does he really need his own bedtime stories, for heaven's sake? Well, yes, apparently, he does. So now as soon as Max starts to snore, I head to Buzz's room, where I find to my delight that he'll even sit through Tracy Kidder's *Mountains Beyond Mountains,* which I've wanted to read for years. And, let's face it, the reading is mostly an excuse to put down the book and snuggle.

As weeks go by, I try out a few other tricks. When I was growing up, my dad, poking fun at himself, used to imitate Akim Tamiroff, in that scene from *For Whom the Bell Tolls* when he keeps saying, "I don't provoke." I teach the boys to say it (getting Tamiroff's gruff accent just right) instead of scratching or biting, and praise them elaborately when they pull it off.

A couple of times, I also try diverting their attention from mayhem with a ritual I've made up, called "the cookie of peace." While they're still lunging at each other, I'll solemnly slice a cookie in half, to put on two plates, which I'll give them as soon as they calm down: a sweet, immediate reward for trying to be civilized.

To my delight, I soon get confirmation that I'm on the right track. Dr. Z. sees Buzz for a checkup and reports that he's "a happier kid. He's less inflamed by his brother. He feels there's more fairness in the family."

Max, unfortunately, doesn't quite share this rosy view. He initially starts teasing Buzz even more fiercely, hissing, "ADD! Retard!" behind my back.

I admonish him. "Max, Buzz is not the bad guy."

"He is, he *is* the bad guy!" he desperately protests.

And then one particularly bad night, after Max throws a piece of macaroni at Buzz that leaves a cheese mark on his new white Dodgers cap, prompting Buzz to hurl a fork across the room at Max's head, I angrily cancel the evening's double reading sessions and stomp off to bed. I'm too troubled to sleep through the night, however, and, five hours later, wake up so thoroughly I figure I might as well try to work. Padding down the hall on the way to my shed, I hear Buzz talking in his room.

He's sitting up, but still asleep.

"Mom, Mom, I have to have my own vision!" he's saying, loudly.

I walk in, sit on his bed, and put my arms around him, making shushing sounds. The moonlight hits our neighbor's cottonwood tree, making the leaves flicker silver through the skylight I used to enjoy when this was still "the family room."

"Mom, my own vision," Buzz repeats. "Wouldn't it be great?"

"Yes, Buzz, that would be great," I say, hugging him. "Absolutely. Your own vision."

I lay him back down, and stay beside him for another ten minutes, making sure he's peaceful.

He's such a precious boy. I so clearly see his goodness.

And then I hear a shrill noise from Max's room. It's his alarm clock, ringing at 2 A.M. My darling Buzz has set a booby trap.

THE PLUM TREES are blooming on the traffic dividers on the mid-April afternoon that I finally head to San Rafael to follow Dr. Z.'s now nearly two-year-old advice to get some coaching on my parenting technique. Marty Edwards, the name I'll use for the psychologist he recommended, is available only on a day when Jack is working, so I go alone, carrying my tape recorder.

Edwards greets me at his office door, looking so tan and virile and relaxed that I doubt he'll be any use at all. Clearly he has never had or even known a child like Buzz. Nonetheless, I walk him through our family history for about fifteen minutes, until I get to my favorite story, about Buzz calling 9-1-1 because I took away his Game Boy. I linger theatrically, suppressing a smile, as I work up to the fabulous punchline, where the cop says: "She took away your what?"

But Edwards doesn't share my mirth. He just looks at me inquiringly, until I elaborate.

"I guess it was kind of a stressful time," I say. "I had this, um, brain tumor. It was benign, so I was really lucky, but I had to have surgery, and right after that, I got thyroid cancer. And, well, then," I add, chuckling, "I broke both my arms. . . ."

I realize only as I say it that I've never summarized that year in quite that way. It seems to make an impression on Edwards. His eyes widen, and he leans closer to my tape recorder, resting on his desk, to slowly intone: "Let the record reflect that my jaw just dropped." Then he spends the next half hour gently grilling me about how I could possibly imagine that those events hadn't made a big difference for Buzz.

I'm not initially sure I want to follow where he's going. *So I had a couple surgeries, big deal: I kept everyone laughing; no one missed a lunch, I think, and only once did I completely forget to pick the kids up from Hebrew school.* But gradually, grudgingly, I start connecting the dots. Buzz's series of extravagant demands—the Karelian bear dog, the Fiji vacation—indeed began during that year that my thoughts were so often turning away from him, toward the mechanics of the upcoming surgery. (*Just how do you open up a skull, anyway?*) And even as I was convincing myself that I was being the best possible, most self-sacrificing, stiff-upper-lipped mom, I know that I reacted to those pleas as if they were personal attacks—*so selfish and inconsiderate!*—while missing the more poignant point.

Early the next morning, while Jack and the boys are still sleeping, I head to my writing shed to do some additional fact-checking, leafing through one of my old diaries, a blue-silk-covered notebook from Chinatown. I've kept journals ever since high school, through all my incarnations, as a student, a newspaper reporter, and a suburban mom. The books now line several of my office shelves. The one I have open chronicles Buzz's tenth year, and now I flip through pages covered in frantic scrawls recording the events leading up to the Game Boy incident. This was just three months, I now see, after the brain scan that found my tumor. I was still having migraines, which by then I was trying to manage with weekly visits to an acupuncturist in Napa, an hour's drive away. He sold me a costly tea—Jack called it "Mom's Vietnamese snake oil"—that stunk up the house for hours after I brewed it.

The journal reminds me how engrossed I was with worrying about the upcoming surgery; how much time I was spending pestering my doctors and prowling the Internet. My memory, which usually likes to put me in the most flattering light, is that I didn't reveal my worries to the kids. Yet right there on the page is a remorseful record of a time I got so mad about their terrible behavior that I made a Nixonesque allusion to how maybe they wouldn't have their mom to kick around in a few more months.

Reading further offers more context. Jack was working overtime, sometimes six days a week . . . Buzz was piling up detentions at school . . . the Buddhist babysitter had just quit . . . and now this jumps out at me: Buzz's 9-1-1 call also took place just two weeks after the afternoon that I first took him to the UCSF clinic, for the tests that led to his diagnosis. One or more of those tests had to be similar to the one that had so panicked me in Colorado.

Did the tests scare Buzz, too? Did he cover up his fear? Come to think of it, why don't I have any record or memory of talking to him about how he felt about being tested and diagnosed? Could I have overlooked that, even as I was dutifully driving him to all those appointments? And what else might I be overlooking now?

As I sit with my open notebook, my previous image of Buzz with the phone in his hand seems to quiver and dissolve. Suddenly, he's no longer my persecutor, the rebel lashing out against a weakened foe, the spoiled symbol of all that's going wrong with American youth, the painfully public proof of how Jack and I have screwed up as parents.

He's just nine years old. He's getting scolded at home, and teased, rejected, and reprimanded every single day at school. His mother is unhappy, her behavior erratic, and he knows just enough about cancer to fear that she might just make good on her threat to disappear.

On top of all this, he has just learned he has something wrong with *his* brain.

He's scared. And he's calling 9-1-1 for help.

HOW OFTEN DO WE ever see each other clearly? Our vision is so blurred by the mists from our pasts that the person we're reacting to is rarely the same person reacting to us.

One of the stories my father loves to tell is about a guy who gets a flat tire on a lonely country road. He has a spare tire in his car, but no jack. He looks up the road, sees a light in a nearby window, and figures he'll ask for help. It's a ten-minute walk, and he starts out thinking, *I'm so glad there's someone there who can help me.* He continues to think along those lines for the next couple minutes, but then it occurs to him: *What if the man in the house doesn't want to help? What if he doesn't trust me? What if he doesn't want to lend his jack? But why shouldn't he? Of course he'll lend his jack! But what if he doesn't? Hey, what kind of guy wouldn't lend a jack?* And so on . . .

By the time the homeowner opens his door, the stranded man is furious. "You can go ahead and shove your damn jack up your ass!" he shouts.

My guess is that my father likes this story so much because he knows how much he sometimes behaves just like that stranded man. And now I see how much Buzz and I have fallen into the same habit toward each other—expecting the worst with every interaction. How can I change course and teach my child that you can't cheat disappointment by counting on it? That it's healthier to cultivate trust?

I don't think that I can explain it with words. But a memory brings me another idea.

Back in Mexico City, I once joined a small group of colleagues for an elegant lunch at the home of the then-U.S. ambassador, John Negroponte. The talk turned to the hard-line U.S. policy toward Cuba, at which point Dudley Althaus, a reporter for the *Houston Chronicle*, asked an offbeat question I'll never forget.

"Why don't you bomb them with love?"

Althaus was suggesting that the United States end its economic embargo and substitute aid that might sell Cuba's people on democracy. He unfortunately failed to change the course of U.S. foreign policy. I can't even remember how Negroponte answered, if he did. But twenty years later, I'm wondering if I can put the strategy to work with Buzz.

So now there's this afternoon when he comes home from school while I'm out working in my shed. He's lost his key, again, so he knocks on the living room window, which of course I don't hear until he knocks so hard the window breaks, strewing glass shards all over the room.

I run to the door, pulse racing, as usual, thinking, *No, not again!? Is he hurt? A trip to the ER? Glass splinters in our hands and butts every time we sit down! Why the hell couldn't he have rung the doorbell, or come around the back? How much is this going to cost?*

But breathing deeply, en route I slow down enough to recognize these thoughts and quiet them before I reach the door, just in time to be able to hear Buzz murmuring something.

"I'm such an idiot!"

And I'm right there to say, "No. No, you're not!"

I'm learning, slowly, to think twice before yelling. Sometimes I even manage not to yell at all. When Buzz melts down, I do my best not to join him. Instead, I often run to microwave the herbal neck pillow my sister Jean sent me, with the insightful advice that I should try to reframe our clashes as dealing with Buzz's feelings—it's the two of us now, against his anger.

The author Toni Morrison says that the best gift a mother can give her child is to light up when he enters the room. I think of all the times my mind was elsewhere, dim to him, and now focus on shining extra brightly. I hug Buzz more often, ignoring his body language that only initially tells me he doesn't want me to come near. I take him out for pizza and don't use the time to grill him about homework. And when Buzz demands that I buy him a wallaby, I put down the latest ADD study I'm reading and sit with him at the computer to look at wallaby pictures (praying I'll find some sort of Health Department ban on them as pets). When he asks me to deliver Chinese food to him at school, I bite back my urge to call him a prince, and say: "The lunch situation is a problem, isn't it? Let's think about what we can do."

But then comes a day when Buzz tells me that Benny Bolansky's mom delivers him a hot lunch every afternoon. At first I refuse to believe it. *Not even in Marin!* Even so, on a subsequent Friday, when Buzz is staying late for a tennis match—a pursuit he earlier fiercely resisted and which I keenly want to encourage—I surprise him by buying a behavior-reinforcing hamburger and milk shake. I place the bag right next to another one on the school counter, which I see is marked "Benny Bolansky."

"It's a special occasion!" I tell the receptionist, who's no doubt drawing some hackneyed conclusion about Jewish mothers. It turns out to be a special occasion every Friday for the rest of the tennis season.

Around this time, I get a chance to talk by phone with Todd Rose's mother, Lyda, who tells me how she figured out the bombing-with-love strategy all by herself. She was just seventeen when Todd was born, and she was initially flummoxed by his bad behavior and all the nasty comments from teachers and relatives. But somehow she managed to turn her attention from her own distress to his. "Todd was dying inside, and for a while, I would never get that," she tells me. "But I finally decided that this kid cannot be attacked everywhere. I have to change at least what happens between him and me."

She began paying much less heed to Todd's teachers and principal, instead coming up with her own plan to help him survive adolescence. When he brought home his report card with all F's and one D, Lyda recalls, "I looked at the D and said, what did you like about this class?"

I'll confess I was relieved to hear later from Todd that Lyda didn't always maintain such exemplary self-control. He remembers, for instance, how she sometimes chased him around the house with a flyswatter. "Kids like me could bring out the child abuse in Mother Teresa," he says generously, adding, "On any given day, if you'd look into our window, you'd see scenes of holy hell. You'd be sure that one of us was going to have to be taken out of there by the authorities, and it wasn't always clear who it should have been." Still, something gradually shifted between mother and son. "Over the long arc of my childhood, I came to appreciate that she was on my side," Rose tells me, adding, "There's no guarantee that a kid will change his life. But when I decided to change, I had a foundation that had been laid down for years and years with no immediate return on investment."

"No immediate return? What about *any* return?" I shoot back.

But I know what he's talking about. Because now that I'm really looking, I can see how much my son—my former nemesis—depends on me. Take the cell phone he bugs me for until I finally relent—guiltily, anxiously, resentfully—on which, one day, I check his list of contacts.

They read, in their redundant entirety:

> Mom
> Home
> Mom

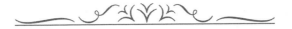

IT'S
CULTURAL

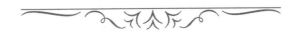

CHAPTER 5

SOCIETY

Attack of the Chronophages

Leisure is a form of that stillness that is the necessary preparation for accepting reality; only the person who is still can hear, and whoever is not still, cannot hear.

JOSEF PIEPER

"THIS IS NOT THE YEAR TO DO CONSTRUCTION ON YOUR HOUSE," warns the woman standing in the front of the synagogue auditorium. She's wearing a tight, floral-patterned silk dress and an air of confident authority.

It's a balmy April evening, with Buzz's bar mitzvah ceremony just five months away. The woman is addressing thirty visibly nervous moms and two cheerful-looking dads sitting in rows of aluminum chairs at a panel on how to prepare for the big event. "This is a sacred year," she tells us. "You need to give yourself permission to experience it."

As I sit in a back row, leafing through lists of caterers, tutoring schedules, sample invitations and programs, I notice that my right eyelid is twitching. It just so happens that two weeks ago, I finally hired a contractor to fix our leaking roof. And as long as he was on board, it seemed reasonable—no, more like *responsible!*—to go ahead and take care of the longstanding termite infestation and, while we were at it, refinish the old wood floors and, oh what the heck, extend the interior roof over the dilapidated front porch to make a new dining room. And move the front door to the other side of the house. "It's the might-as-wells that'll get ya," laughed the loan officer when I called to try to get our equity line increased.

Back in the early 1980s, my reporter friend Pete Carey warned me to beware of "chronophages"—the "time-eaters" that get in the way of more important things, like working. And here I've invited a swarm of new chronophages into my life at the worst possible moment. Seven months into this would-be sacred year, this year I've pledged to spend paying attention to what's truly important, my brain is crammed with details about town permits and paint colors and contractors' fees, and sixty-three options for "flush mount" ceiling fixtures, not to mention all the extra consulting work I'll need to do to help pay for it all. I'm running way overbudget—not only in money and time, but in mental resources.

In the synagogue auditorium, another woman has gotten up to speak. She's explaining how, during the bar mitzvah year, families are expected to attend, at minimum, a half a dozen Friday night and Saturday morning Shabbat services. *Sure, no problem!* I think to myself.

Yet in fact, that's exactly the problem, isn't it? Every one of the commitments now threatening to overwhelm me seemed like such a good idea at the time. It all started as soon as Buzz began to edge out of his daily-crisis mode, giving me the wherewithal to notice all the other signs of looming entropy that I'd previously ignored. The house has been a mess for years. Fixing it up would make a public announcement that order had been restored at last, that our home was somewhere you'd no longer expect to see someone, like me, for instance, running out the front door, yelling, "I can't take it anymore!"

Besides, the extra work I've taken on to pay the contractor, on top of some overdue therapy bills, is not only financially necessary, but also so refreshingly meaningful and worldly, after all my narrow focus on Buzz and myself. Several months of cultivating contacts has paid off with a sudden bounty of offers, which is why I'm now simultaneously helping to write a new "conservation atlas" for the Nature Conservancy, drafting a speech on green-energy investments for a

Silicon Valley billionaire, and consulting on a new Web site for Google.org, the philanthropic arm of Google. How, really, am I supposed to turn any of this down? Especially considering I've already said *yes, yes, yes!*?

Even so, ever since the afternoon that the wrecking crew arrived, bringing its daily hammering and the fine coat of dust on the kitchen counters, I've noted an uptick in the chronic frequency of lost keys, sunglasses, earring backs, socks, and vital documents, as well as complaints from family members and friends whose calls I haven't returned. I got ticketed just last week for rolling past the same stop sign at which I'd been ticketed just two weeks earlier. Worst of all, after more than half a year of intensive research and tests and meds and insights galore, I'm *still* blowing up at Buzz. Especially when he takes forever (it sure *seems* deliberate) to put on his socks when he's already late for school, or willfully (I think) fails to write down his homework assignments or bring home his agenda, or pounds on Max (granted, usually after Max teases him).

"An explosive outburst . . . occurs when the cognitive demands being placed upon a person outstrip that person's capacity to respond adaptively," writes the Harvard psychologist Ross Greene. Greene is writing about explosive *children,* but as life becomes more cognitively taxing, he might as well include their parents.

If I've learned anything by now, it's that kids like Buzz do best with parents who aren't having tantrums right back at them, or even frantically checking e-mail every five minutes—parents able to listen closely and explain things patiently and repeatedly. Yet this sort of self-control so easily eludes me when I'm in my default mode of scrambling around in frustration over projects left up in the air. Ever since I moved from Brazil to the multitasking U.S. suburbs, I've become like a car so plastered over with bumper stickers that I can no longer see out the windshield. *"I Brake for Fevers." "I Brake for Early School-Day Release Due to Parent-Teacher Conferences." "I Brake for Any Potential Income-Generating Activity." "I Brake for Regular Cancer Follow-up Blood Tests, Brain Scans, and Appointments." "I Brake for All Calls and E-Mails from Jack, My Parents, Siblings, Consulting Clients,*

Various Close Women Friends . . . and Now, Of Course, Also the Con-
tractor, Who Seems Like He Calls Every Half Hour." . . .

A story is told in recovery groups about a woman who keeps walk-ing down the same street and falling into the same hole, until she fi-nally learns to walk down another street. When it comes to mastering my attention, I suppose I've at least reached the point where I can see the hole and know I tend to fall in it. Still, here I am again, with my nose on the pavement.

This, in fact, is a trademark danger of serious distraction: to flee from boredom straight into frantic overcommitment. What's new today, however, is that it's no longer just folks like Buzz and me who're driven to these extremes. The rest of the world is quickly catching up.

In the time I've spent lost in these thoughts, sitting on my alumi-num chair, a third woman has stood up to explain about how each bar mitzvah candidate is expected to come up with a philanthropic "mitzvah project" this year. I already know that most of the other kids in Buzz's class are well under way with tutoring disadvantaged chil-dren, caring for injured wildlife, or raising money to send to Darfur. Yet Buzz has yet to offer a plan. I take out my notebook to write my-self a reminder to think harder about how I might help get him moti-vated, then slip from my seat as quietly as I can, with a sheepish grin for the three panelists and the more than half of the audience mem-bers who turn their heads unsmilingly to track my early exit. Time is running out, after all, and before my year is up—like, starting *tonight*—I need to understand more clearly why I and nearly everyone else I know these days seem so hopelessly overwhelmed, and if there's any hope of a cure.

THE SCREEN ABOVE the receptionist's desk at Google.org in San Francisco displays Internet searches, in real time, taking place all over the world. Pulses of acquisitiveness, anxiety, and curiosity flash by in Roman, Arabic, and Chinese alphabets: "Pottery Barn . . . Aleve . . . *juegosjuegos* . . . Zingerman's delicatessen . . . U.S. Open 2006 . . . I wanna be there when you go insane lyrics . . . *ilhas desertas* . . . Jack Black college . . . caloric restriction age-related disease . . . Airforce forms 357 . . ."

I've been invited here to help out with a meeting on "messaging," which is how many contemporary PR people refer to PR. With two weeks having passed since my soul-searching at the bar mitzvah preparation panel, it might be reasonable to think that I'd have made some progress in paring down my list of commitments so as to culti-vate more calm and focus, and zero in on this year's priority: my quest to understand and help my son. Alas, that would be wrong.

I want to figure out how to be a better parent. I want to write a graceful, helpful book. I also want to work for Google, the coolest company around. I've already had such a great time dropping the name into conversations. ("Speaking of food, I ate the most amazing noodle dish the other day—*at Google!*")

Still, it's not just status that has lured me here, but fear. Because I can't stop reading the news, I've become seriously preoccupied by the risks accumulating from antibiotic-resistant bacteria, SARS, the North Korean nuclear threat, Osama bin Laden, and, always, more than any-thing, global warming. I worry to what even I know is an unhealthy extreme about Chinese coal plants, Exxon's lobbyists, and the threat to global food supplies. Sometimes, just before going to sleep, I'll be reading some article about rising sea levels and try to get Jack to talk it over with me.

"Isn't there something we should be doing?" I'll ask. "I mean, like moving to higher ground, or learning about indoor agriculture?"

"It'll be all right," he'll murmur, turning back to his crossword puzzle, even as I'll insist: "*What* will? *How?*"

Here at Google.org, however, folks are not only willing to think about global warming and other major threats but are actually trying to do something, as I happily reflect, while I follow the twenty-something receptionist into the wood-paneled conference room. I was hooked as soon as I read a *New York Times* article announcing the philanthropy's plans to tackle not only energy reform, but developing-world poverty and disease—all at once! *Those are my kind of people!*

In the conference room, the meeting is already under way, with about a dozen seemingly twenty-something people focused on figuring out how to describe Google.org's wide-ranging endeavors for its Web site and other PR materials. Drafts of the content are projected onto one of the walls, and people interrupt one another to call out wordsmithing ideas, which a slim young woman dressed in black types on her laptop. A screen on the opposite wall, meanwhile, displays the giant face of a young man joining us by teleconference. He's chewing on something, which I guess is lunch, assuming he's in our time zone. The young man next to me is also eating—from a big, redolent meat-and-noodle dish—while typing away, and periodically grabbing and staring at his cell phone. In fact, as I now notice, every person in the room is alternating between participating in the discussion and focusing on his or her laptop and/or buzzing and/or vibrating phone or pager, checking e-mails, text-messaging, and doing Internet searches. In the years since I left the newsroom and stayed out of the traditional workforce, the whole concept of work has apparently changed. I've read that white-collar workers today get interrupted on average every two minutes, but until now I assumed it couldn't be true.

After an hour, I'm starting to feel so left out that I check my own cell phone. There's just one message, from Jack, who wants to know what's for dinner.

Twenty-first-century information technology is particularly dangerous catnip for boredom-averse novelty-junkies like me, in that it offers a constant flow of external temptations to add to those we come up with all by ourselves. It shouldn't be any wonder, however, that the rest of the world is also vulnerable. As I've been learning, in between all my daily distractions, all humans are novelty-lovers, to varying degrees. The trait harks back to all those years that our hunter-gatherer ancestors spent on the savannah, where newness was rare and often meant great danger (a new snake!) or great reward (a new berry!). We've evolved so that dopamine, that key neurotransmitter, greets each fresh stimulus with a chemical *zing!* while a tiny, mid-brain structure called the superior colliculus prompts our gaze to shift and head to turn.

The difficulty comes in trying to adapt this ancient system to a world of nonstop novelty, with considerable social pressure to distinguish between fourteen kinds of salad greens, and keep up with the latest iPhone iteration, and be polite to all sorts of people who, thanks to technology, have an expanding number of ways to contact us out of the blue. One survey I read said nearly half of all information workers will respond to an e-mail within sixty minutes of receiving it—a self-defeating strategy that, again, must owe to the caveman years in which humans could live to a ripe old age knowing no more than about fifty other people, and couldn't afford to diss any of them.

As I look around the meeting room at Google.org, I marvel at how these mostly obsolete urges, combined with a finite number of waking hours, keep driving us to "multitask," despite increasing evidence that it's a losing game. Scientists have shown that our brains actually can't do more than one thing at once: we multitask by toggling between endeavors, leading to a lot of wasted time, errors, and stress. Way back in 2002—and you can just imagine how much worse it's since become—the National Highway Traffic Safety Administration estimated at least 955 deaths and 240,000 accidents annually were caused by drivers talking on cell phones. Some years later, researchers revealed that workers dividing attention between phone calls and e-mails temporarily lose more than twice the IQ points as they would if they smoked dope.

What's more, it's not just smarts we're sacrificing by striving to do it all—we're also losing perspective. Just a couple weeks ago, while I was working as part of a team on that speech for the Silicon Valley billionaire, one of his assistants, profusely apologizing, excused himself for a day—to attend the birth of his first child. Late that night, he sent a long e-mail from the delivery room, where he was still worrying over details in the speech, which wasn't due, in any case, for a couple of weeks. Call him anytime, he urged us, adding, once more, "my apologies for skipping out."

Google, of course, is the eye of this hurricane of getting and spending and keeping in touch, a particularly American way of life that the psychiatrist Peter C. Whybrow has compared to the mental disorder known as mania: a "frenetic chase . . . that begins with a joyous sense of excitement and high productivity but escalates into reckless pursuit, irritability, and confusion, before cycling down into depression." I know I should keep far away from it all, like an alcoholic shunning even one drink, but I have to admit that a certain amount of stress and chaos feels so invigoratingly familiar. Throughout my childhood, I watched my father invent his own emergencies, swinging between spending sprees hailed with an exuberant "Hang the expense!"—and remorseful anxiety, ushered in with a groan of "It's *erev mechula!*": Yiddish for "the eve of bankruptcy." I feel right at home in this meeting room, where everyone seems to be racing to put out several fires at once.

Over three afternoon meetings, we all sort-of listen to a parade of speakers who come in to describe campaigns to spur production of plug-in hybrid cars, make renewable energy cheaper than coal, create middle-class jobs in the developing world, and improve detection of emerging epidemics. The only problem, as we try to figure out how to describe all these efforts, is that many of them haven't yet begun. As silly as I feel about doing it, I keep asking the same question over and over again: "So what exactly are you doing?" I get a lot of nods in response, but few clear answers.

After the third meeting, the staff employee who hired me walks me back out to the lobby, looking exasperated. Our special bond is that we're both over thirty. When we first met, several months ago, she told me: "I think you can offer some clarity here." At the time, it struck me as delightfully ironic. But not anymore. I have seen the future, I guess, and it's not a friendly place for a clinically distracted mom trying to cope with a clinically distracted child.

I do a little bit more work—*for Google!*—over the next few weeks, but remain on the outskirts of the action, whatever the action is.

BY MID-JUNE, with my self-imposed deadline fast approaching for solving my attention problems, getting Buzz in better shape, and finishing my book, I am finally ready to admit that I need help to lighten my load of distractions. Luckily, this is when I get to spend a week with my mother and psychiatrist sister, Jean, at a trendy vegetarian spa on the Mexican border. Despite all I've learned from the interviews and reading I've fit between my "messaging" and speech-writing, I'm still trying, clumsily, to multitask: we're purportedly here to relax and celebrate my mother's eightieth birthday, but I'm also seeking to defray our expenses by giving a couple of talks on writing to the other guests, while also checking e-mail every few hours in the spa's always-crowded Internet room, to keep up with my consulting projects and badger Jack about not letting the boys play video games all day long. In whatever time remains, I take early morning hikes on desert mountain trails, lift weights, learn tai chi, and eat organic salads and spicy soups. There's tennis, salsa, cardio-boxing, swimming, and meditation—and I want, as usual, to do it all.

On our third afternoon, Jean and I and a dozen other women, our average age roughly fifty-five, attend a "life coaching" workshop led by a muscular guy in his twenties. We spend the first ten minutes of time rolling our eyes at one another, before we walk out.

"Was that a joke, or what?" Jean asks, as we stop by the dining hall to fill glasses with herbal ice tea, which we take outside to a wooden picnic table under an olive tree.

"Right, I think we could probably do a better job for each other, don't you think?" I ask. "Like, less studly, but more experienced?"

Jean already knows why I need life-coach advice, because I've been complaining about my overloaded agenda to her for months now, during our twice-weekly phone calls. With just an hour to spare before her facial, she launches in, bluntly as usual: "You know, you don't have ADD. You're just trying to do too much."

"Maybe I'm trying to do too much *because* I have ADD," I say.

"Write down your list," Jean tells me, and I obediently open my notebook. The strapping life coach has suggested we do this, describing our various time-sinks to see where we might be able to cut back.

It takes me about ten minutes to identify twenty items, with the hungriest chronophages first. They start, of course, with Buzz.

After doing so well for the first months of our special year, he has faltered in recent weeks, with teachers complaining about him zoning out, and lots of reprimands for chewing gum and talking back. He even got suspended just before the school year ended, following a fistfight with a boy Buzz claimed started it by calling him "Jewy." (Jack and I were prepared to hate the boy and his anti-Semitic family, until we met the exhausted-looking parents at school and learned that Buzz's combatant also has ADD, but hadn't taken his meds that day. We ended up trading notes on therapists, books, and support groups.)

Max, meanwhile, seems to be fighting all the harder for my increasingly wandering focus. "WAR!! What is it GOOD FOR??" he shouts, while doing his math homework at the kitchen table. Catching my eye, he asks, "Why do acorns have Xs on them? Are we going to have World War III? Would there have been a Hitler if there hadn't been a Christ? What would happen to liquid if there were no gravity?"

How I wish that my children could just hang on until I find a more convenient time to spend with them. But they're not interested in waiting around for quality time; they want what they can get right now, and when they don't get it, and, increasingly, even when they do, there are always those gadgets: Xboxes, PSPs, Game Boys, and Internet social networking sites, where the cognitive rewards, with flashing graphics and noise, are immediate and addictive, and where I fear that, if allowed, they would cheerfully waste whole days and nights, like those little lab rats in the experiments in which the rats ignore hunger and thirst to keep pressing a bar to get cocaine. Todd Rose says that I'm too anxious about the amount of time my kids spend hypnotized by technology. "Back in the days when the printing press was first invented, people worried that books would rob us of our storytelling abilities," he reminds me.

I realize I may seem silly, single-handedly trying to ward off the New Millennium, but as usual, I'm keeping files of news reports supporting my fears about the erosion of our concentration, conversations, and courtesy. They inspire me to keep shouldering the major

modern parental chronophage of actively offering substitutes: shut-
tling the boys off to after-school activities, reading books to them if
they won't read them themselves, and spending far too much time
nagging. Jack and I have issued a rule that electronic stimulation is
limited to watching *The Simpsons* as a family on weekdays, plus two
hours of games each weekend day. The kids have complied with this
about twice, but I keep trying to enforce it, often hiding TV cords
and gadgets, and then, alas, nearly just as often forgetting where I've
put them and having to waste even more time searching, or having to
buy new ones. One summer, after reading reports of the alarming
"nature deficit" supposedly adding to our children's attention deficits,
I went to the extreme of dragging my sons to a cattle ranch, where by
prearrangement with the open-minded ranchers, the three of us fed
cows, dug ditches, and cleaned the chicken coop to earn our keep. In
the afternoons, Buzz played by the creek, and once ventured out in a
boat where he proudly caught a large bass we cooked for dinner. At
night, I read *To Kill a Mockingbird* aloud. We were back in the olden
days. The kids fought less. I wanted to stay there forever. After the
third day, however, the two of them gravitated toward the ranchers'
kitchen to play on the floor with the cats. And there they stayed,
mutely refusing to do more chores. "They're *indoor* boys," the frown-
ing ranch wife observed.

Lucky, blessed, and grateful as I feel about being a mother, I also
frequently resent the hell out of how much of my time my kids demand. And I know I'm not alone here. Modern parents report that
we're spending more hours per week with our children than did parents forty years ago, even as we confess that it makes us roughly as
happy as doing housework.

I suspect distraction has something to do with this, as well. Many
of these extra hours we say we're spending with our kids are hours
we're necessarily also doing something else, even something as simple as driving them somewhere. And as I've come to understand, I'm
most content in the rare moments when I'm able to do just one thing
at once, and *least* content when I'm worrying that we've run out of
toilet paper, while trying to break up a fight, while waiting on hold for

the gas-company billing department. (Which I suppose is technically spending time with the kids.)

Which brings me back to my list.

Just looking at those twenty items makes me feel exhausted. How did I ever convince myself I could carry them all, without screwing up in some major way?

After all the caregiving hours for Buzz and Max and the minimal attention I can sometimes scrounge for Jack comes the time dedicated to working on, at last count, three part-time consulting projects, my supposedly full-time book research, and the monthly column I write for an environmental journal.

"Well, you obviously can't cut any of these," Jean says, drawing her perfectly manicured fingernail from #1 to #8.

My parents are also in the can't-eliminate category—I call them every day, and visit twice a month—as is, of course, grocery shopping and laundry and picking stray popcorn kernels up from the floor, with the recent addition of a few hours a week to supervise and assist in the out-of-control remodeling project. Next comes the shamefully paltry but soul-feeding amount of philanthropic/community activity I've taken on: giving blood, dropping off meals at a homeless shelter, and serving on Buzz's middle school parent-teacher advisory council. And last: the profound solace of time snatched from the jaws of domesticity to spend with an assortment of women friends.

Hey, come to think of it, *everything* is in the can't-eliminate category!

Jean frowns at my list, as I gloomily watch a blackbird swoop down to nibble at an abandoned bran muffin crumbling on a nearby table. I've moved on from reproaching myself for trying to do too much to reproaching myself for not doing enough to make the most of this "sacred year" in which Buzz is gearing up for manhood. The bar mitzvah preparations have so much potential significance to savor, not least the relationships Buzz and I have begun with his three terrific-male-role-model tutors: Cantor David, Rabbi Michael, and his regular, twice-weekly teacher, Jay. Early on I confessed to each of them, in turn, how apprehensive I am about possibly expecting too much from a kid who is already struggling at school. Their answers offered variations on the theme that this particular expectation is just what Buzz needs. Cantor David also confidently assured me that he has shepherded "thousands" of kids through the process and hasn't lost one yet, while Rabbi Michael took Buzz out for ice cream to coax him to think a little more about his mitzvah project, and Jay has been unfailingly steady and patient. *What have I done for these wonderful men, in return? Shouldn't I have cooked something for them by now?*

I also know there's a lot more magic that I could be mining from each planning ritual along the way. As Buzz and I pick out invitations, party food, and clothes, we've begun to imagine people reading, eating, and watching, as the bar mitzvah vision becomes ever more real. Yet too often, in the hubbub of my days, these potentially meaningful moments get short-shrifted down to mere additions to my to-do list, and more reasons for squabbling with Buzz. His penchant for pricey demands is flaring up again: he's still pouting over my refusal to order the $400 deluxe gold-ink invitations he fell in love with on the Internet, and pestering for a post–bar mitzvah party in Hawaii.

"Buzz," I finally said, in exasperation the other day, "what if you had to choose between a Lakers theme for the party and curing guinea worm infestations in Africa?"

"Could I do half-and-half?" he promptly replied.

His latest Karelian-bear-doggish campaign, which began shortly after he saw Daniel Craig as James Bond in *Casino Royale,* is that he wants to rent a white tuxedo for the bar mitzvah day. My dad blew a gasket when I mentioned it. "What does your rabbi say about that?!" he demanded. I haven't asked; I don't need to. *The white tux is out of the question; even I can see that. . . .*

Jean rouses me back to the present, tapping her fingernail on the page. "Some of these have got to go," she says. "What about this parent-teacher group?"

"Oh, I can't cut that!" I blurt out.

She looks at me searchingly. "You need to look at that reaction," she says, in a tone a bit too clinical for comfort.

"It would be humiliating to drop out, even though I hate it and it's a useless waste of time," I protest. "I'm signed on for three years. This is the last year. It's just one afternoon a month."

As I consider Jean's advice, nonetheless, a chill runs down my back. What if people think I'm a flake? That I've let them down? That I'm actually *not* the fantasy mom who keeps all her professional and social commitments while running a reproach-proof home? I do realize other people probably aren't thinking about me half as much as I'm thinking about their thinking about me. And there's so much I could do with those three hours a month. . . .

Jean sighs theatrically and moves on. She has already skipped over the item that says "exercise—7 hours a week," because she and I share the view that a reasonable amount of aerobic activity is a necessity: our only hedge against otherwise rapid deterioration of our minds as well as our bodies. But she pauses at the entry that says, "North 24th"—the name of the nonfiction writers' group that I joined about a year ago. The ten of us meet twice a month to comment on one another's work over coffee and scones, sharing grievances, triumphs, and answers to all sorts of urgent, arcane questions like whether I can let Buzz eat a maraschino cherry wrapped in a cocktail napkin and forgotten in my purse overnight. (Surprisingly, yes! At least according to the consensus.) Our strictest rule is that we always start with praise. If someone hands in a rambling first draft, filled with clichés and non sequiturs, each one of these talented women will manage to unearth its hidden gems. I've only recently summoned the nerve to start submitting my own rambling drafts, prompting my friends to respond with the best advice I've ever received about writing or anything else. "Slow down," they say. "And keep going."

"You've got to look harder at some of these things that aren't providing you with income," Jean says.

"I know," I say. "Let's look at the next one."

After twenty more minutes, we've gone through the list, and I've refused to cut a single item.

"Are we wasting our time here?" Jean asks, not so gently.

Initially I fear she's right. Yet as the weeks go by, with the memory of my impossible list stuck in my mind, something shifts. Some changes happen by attrition: consulting jobs end, and I don't take on new ones. I also make a few hard choices: I eventually do quit the parent-teacher council and ease up just a bit on trying to enforce that electronic-stimulation rule, which was a laughingstock in any case. I also work harder at getting Jack to do more of the busywork, such as taking the kids to the dentist on his day off.

In time, my heightened sensitivity to chronophages helps me get better at fending them off. Each time I'm tempted to respond to an e-mailed chain letter or forwarded YouTube video or aimless Facebook entry, I try to keep in mind an old World War II slogan the federal government put on posters to discourage unnecessary travel: "Is Your Trip Necessary?"

When the Internet connection in my writing shed breaks down, I don't fix it, which means I have to walk back into the house to check e-mail. I also train myself so that whenever I get an impulse, while involved in some task, to jump up and do something else, I write it down on a sheet of paper instead, and put the paper in a manila file, marked "Soon!"

In time, all of these efforts add up, improving my focus enough to help me spot other potential time-wasters. Eventually, I even find myself doing some things without trying to do something else at the same time.

At home, I start paying a little more attention to food, after so many years of harried takeout. On Friday nights, I cook dinner and light candles to welcome the Sabbath. I bless the bread and put my hands on my sons' heads to bless them, too. The boys always laugh, but they remind me if I ever forget to do it.

OKAY, so much for good intentions. Like a dummy, I'm trying to multitask *again,* half-listening to the news hour on the radio while driving and also attempting to supervise four kids in the carpool on the way to Hebrew school. It's a weekly, unfailing blood-pressure boost that I've come to refer to as "the Tuesday Death March." Like so many of my other commitments, this carpool initially seemed like a good idea, mainly because I wasn't paying enough attention to the fact that it requires three separate pickup stops en route to the synagogue, half an hour from home, and includes a couple kids who are at least as badly behaved as my own. Buzz sits in the front seat, which he'll still jerk back occasionally to ram whoever's sitting behind him, while Max is in the back next to Andy, age five, who sits in his booster seat, intermittently screaming with joy or rage, and his brother Stephen, ten, whose specialty is noisy farts that prompt everyone to roll down windows and howl.

All four of these children reliably unite to harangue me to stop on the way to school for snacks, which I'm usually too late or too furious at them to buy. Today, however, the quality of their behavior has risen to a few degrees short of abysmal, so I've yielded and swerved into a drive-through to pick up milk shakes.

As I swerve out, Stephen yells: "There's a booger on the seat!"

Andy is bouncing up and down, laughing hysterically.

"I didn't do it!" Max shouts, before anyone can accuse him.

"He sure did!" Buzz yells, throwing his baseball cap at him.

"HE did," Max cries. "He always blames me!"

I pull over to the side of the road, a waste of five more minutes we can't spare. But it's not safe to keep driving with this chaos in the car. Stephen is flopping around as if trying to flee from the evil-looking glob on the seat back facing him.

Attempting a diversionary tactic, I take a tissue out of my purse, snarling, "I'm taking this to a DNA lab, so if I were the one who did it, I'd want to start talking, now!"

No one falls for this, but at least they stop yelling. We arrive at the synagogue with spilled milk shake all over the backseat and Max in tears—and Buzz now ten minutes late for his private bar mitzvah tutoring which I've so skillfully coordinated to coincide with the other kids' classes. I grab Buzz's arm, barking pickup instructions to the three other boys, then drag my son to the room in the upstairs library where Jay, a seventy-something scholar in suspenders, shiny shoes, and an old green fedora, has been waiting. He looks up at us, and then his eyes drift toward the clock on the wall.

"Sorry, sorry, sorry," I murmur, and as Buzz jerks free to run to the bathroom, I seize the moment to add in a whisper, *"He's a little ADD!"*

Jay's eyes widen softly as his only reply.

I choose a chair near the window, intending to spend the next half hour reading some of the research studies I've printed out for just such spare moments. But ten minutes later, the printouts remain unread, as I lean back to absorb the strange tranquility that has settled in the room. Buzz, wearing a yarmulke, is tilting toward Jay, chanting ancient Hebrew blessings that join his squeaky tenor with the older man's low growl.

The Torah is read each year from start to finish, with a new installment every Saturday morning. The bar mitzvah candidate's job is to lead the Sabbath service, reciting several prayers plus a passage of his choice from the day's Torah portion and a related haftarah portion from the prophets.

Buzz's Torah portion is from Deuteronomy, the part where the Israelites have reached the Promised Land. Moses is telling them the rules they must follow in their new home, and warning of the awful fates awaiting those who don't comply. Locusts. Hemorrhoids. Blindness. Robbery. Fear. Dismay. Death. From all this grim material, however, Buzz has found and chosen twelve upbeat lines describing how God will reward compliance. His choice heartens me, like a bright view of his own future.

"Blessed shall you be in the city, and blessed shall you be in the country," Buzz sings, haltingly sounding out the Hebrew letters. "The Lord will give you abounding prosperity in the issue of your womb, the offspring of your cattle, and the produce of your soil. . . ."

"Very good!" Jay tells him periodically, with more than a hint of surprise in his tone. I've been trying to manage Jay's expectations with frequent complaints about how little Buzz is studying at home. Yet my son seems to be memorizing the passage as we watch. His eyes shine with Jay's praise, and his voice rises more boldly. I no longer see any resemblance to the boy who called me an "asshole" after I dragged him out of bed on the third try this morning.

I sit to the side, out of this loop, reflecting on how I've read that the Kabbalah, Jewish mystic lore, refers to the bar mitzvah as "a science of knots to undo," the main knot, naturally, being the one between a boy and his mother. There's such power in this ancient, public test, with its communal expectation that a child behave like a man in front of his elders, at such a fragile and pivotal time of his life. I picture Buzz as the Jewish equivalent of a young Masai warrior, going out to kill his first lion, or a naked Amazonian Indian youth, his face painted for a night of dancing and chanting. And I'm drawn into the moment in a way that makes the time in this small, hot room suddenly so much more than one more item to cross off on my list. I wouldn't call it leisure, but it's certainly stillness, and it comes with a comforting thought: *Maybe not a sacred* year. *But surely a few sacred minutes. . . .*

CHAPTER 6

EDUCATION

The Rules of Engagement

*It is little short of a miracle that modern
methods of instruction have not already completely
strangled the holy curiosity of inquiry.*

ALBERT EINSTEIN

"HEY, PUT THAT AWAY!" I HISS.

Buzz sticks his tongue out at me, as he proceeds to plug in the earphones of his new iPod. It's the one I recently bought to help him memorize his bar mitzvah chants, recorded by our synagogue's cantor, but which instead he has loaded with graphic songs, including one called "My Dick."

This is so embarrassing. We've traveled all the way to Boston's Brigham and Women's Hospital, an affiliate of Harvard University Medical School, to watch Todd Rose teach a special summer school class on brain science to inner-city teenagers working at the hospital. We've all just taken our seats at school desks in the front row of the windowless classroom, and, unlike Buzz, the dozen students seem expectant and tuned in.

Rose walks briskly to the front of the room, looking every bit a missionary, with his close-cropped hair and white button-down shirt. He's just about to launch into his talk when he shoots a glance at Buzz. Without mentioning the iPod, he simply introduces us by name—lassoing my son's attention with one of the oldest tricks in the book.

"Katherine and Buzz are visiting us today all the way from California," he says, in his race-track delivery, adding, "Katherine is actually my parole officer."

Buzz laughs along with the other students. Then he puts his iPod in his pocket, where it stays for the rest of the next hour.

I've brought Buzz along with me on this research trip with the hope that meeting Rose will help light his inner fire, get him caring about something, anything, besides his Xbox, the Dodgers, the Lakers, and overpriced shoes. He didn't need convincing: he loves adventures, airplanes, restaurant meals, and maybe more than anything, the fact that his brother Max wasn't invited. Now, to my delight, I notice that he's listening intently, as Rose regales the class with a story that not only borders on the obscene but, as far as I can tell, has little if anything to do with neuroscience. He's telling how, as a boy growing up in rural Utah, he once peed on a cattle-proof fence.

"I mean, don't ever try that!" he says, shaking with laughter. "I got the shock of my life!"

Darting back to his laptop, he flips through his PowerPoint slides. There's a cartoon picture of a kid sticking a knife into an electric socket and a photograph of a boy about to slide down a giant ramp into the ocean. Rose, chuckling, tells story after story, often interrupting himself before he can get to the punchline. He talks so fast that you're compelled to pay close attention, even if you aren't already hypnotized by the way he's racing around the room. A walking emoticon, he'll stop suddenly to imitate a monkey in attack mode, or wave an imaginary baseball bat, checking himself in mid-swing to illustrate how someone controls a reflex. Entertaining as he is, his earnest purpose soon grows clear: he's building an inviting scaffold—think jungle gym—on which to hang abstract concepts about impulsivity and self-restraint. The kids are drawn in by his stories, only later realizing the good-for-you insights they offer about temperament and behavior, and the reasons people succeed or fail. By then, story and insight are melded together, in the way, as Rose will later tell me, that we all learn best.

Rose calls this "evidence-based teaching," since there's so much research confirming that a sense of excitement and relevance, stories and mystery, and, probably more than anything else, a student's connection with his teacher, powerfully influence how well he learns. "No one's brain can form memories—learn, that is—without being engaged in some way," Rose says. "Your heart has to beat just a little bit faster; your pupils dilate almost microscopically. Your brain has to be *aroused,* which sounds suggestive, but really just means you have to care."

This emotional connection, so important to all students, is both more essential and harder to achieve for kids like Buzz, who're at constant risk of tuning out or acting up. Many U.S. school administrators already know this, which is why they talk so much about "engagement." Nonetheless, throughout the country—including in my own supposedly progressive West Coast suburb, where we moved, after all, for the schools—the vast majority of classrooms still chug along under the old, factory-inspired model, with students expected to memorize information while sitting quietly at their desks. The "No Child Left Behind" Act, with its emphasis on standardized tests, has reinforced this rote-learning approach, which is famously bad for boys in general. At this writing, only 65 percent of American boys, compared to 72 percent of girls, are graduating from high school. If your child is clinically distracted, however, the odds that the system will fail him are even worse, leading to many more suspensions, expulsions, and dropouts than with other children. Researchers report that up to 60 percent of children with ADD will get suspended, and as many as 40 percent will drop out of school.

As a parent in this predicament, your options boil down to three: fight the system, find an alternative, or face the predictably bleak consequences.

"I DON'T WANT TO ruin your weekend, but—" the voice on the phone begins.

It's a Friday afternoon, and I'm in my writing shed, chewing sug-
arless tangerine gum, agonizing over a clunky first draft, and long-
ing, as always, for distraction, although I wouldn't have ordered this
one. The voice belongs to Buzz's English teacher, who is graciously
taking time to let me know he hasn't turned in a major assignment
due today, which—it's news to me—he should have been working
on for the past week. The instruction was to interview someone,
preferably a parent, about prejudice. Buzz hasn't even gotten started.
His teacher isn't sure why that is, but, again, graciously—and maybe
also because I've met with her three times by now to plead for
understanding—she offers Buzz a reprieve as long as he can do the
work this weekend.

Whenever I ask Buzz if he has homework these days, he tells me
that he already finished it at school. He won't write assignments in
his agenda, even when Xbox time depends on it, and there is little
else he cares about, other than food, which I'm not yet ready to with-
hold.

So when Buzz comes home this afternoon, I leave my shed,
microwave him a plate of leftover spaghetti, and spend the next half
hour arguing, bribing, threatening, and pulling out the TV cord and
hiding it, before finally convincing him to get started. The two of us,
I'm well aware, are trapped in an all-but-senseless system: even as
U.S. teachers are piling on ever more homework, research has shown
it doesn't measurably improve academic achievement in grade school,
although it *can* sour kids' attitudes toward school, and increase conflict between them and their parents. I should probably spend more
time complaining about this to Buzz's principal, who already thinks
I'm a crank. But in the short term, I just don't want him to fail. It
drives me crazy that I have to work this hard. And it makes me so sad
to think of all the worried mothers who don't even have this option.

Finally, he sits down in front of the computer. He smooths out
the crumpled blue instruction sheet we've fished from the bottom of
his backpack—a trove of ancient cookie crumbs, leaking pens, un-
signed permission slips, and unwashed gym shorts—and starts typing fast.

"Wait. Hold on," I interrupt. "You haven't done the interview, have you?"

"Yes, I have," Buzz says, eyes locked on the screen.

"Who'd you interview? It's supposed to be a parent."

"I interviewed Tomás Mooger."

"Tomás Mooger?"

"Yeah. I met him in a chat room."

"You met Tomás Mooger in a chat room?"

Perhaps a better mother would have nourished this creative impulse by drawing Buzz out about his intriguing invented character. *Why the Latin influence? What inspired the "Mooger"?* My long-range plan, of course, is to be that better mother. But right now, I'm worn out and impatient and, as so often is the case come 5 P.M., still haven't a clue what I'm cooking for dinner. So instead, I grit my teeth and tell Buzz he must *follow the rules,* feeling a pang for the teachers who must try to manage thirty or more kids per class, including three or four who are equally resistant. It takes a full, grueling hour of our time, but through sheer force of nagging, I eventually get Buzz to interview me and finish his homework (which the next day he'll forget to hand in).

Buzz is blessedly less troubled and angry these days, but he still clearly hates school. I suspect one big reason for this is he hasn't yet found his "bliss"—the passion that might help make all that drudgery bearable.

A year ago, I sat with Buzz in his psychiatrist's office as Dr. Z. asked him what he most liked to do.

"Eat," Buzz replied.

"Something doesn't add up here," Dr. Z. later told me. "A mind as bright and lively as his should have found a place by now in the world of books and ideas. He's a boy who's very bright but not engaged. There's some interference."

Maybe it's simply his dopamine glitch. People like Buzz—and me, and Todd Rose in our past lives—can easily get branded as lazy, because the carrots and sticks that get most people moving just don't work as well with us. We need bigger, sweeter carrots and humongous, scary sticks.

I suppose I've been lucky in this respect. I got hooked on the carrots of glory and riches at age eleven, when Archie Comics sent me a $5 check for an essay I wrote about our pet miniature schnauzer, while the early stick of my father's volatile temper was soon enough replaced by my terror of missing a newspaper deadline.

My younger son, Max, leans toward my own anxiously motivated style. He does his homework the minute he returns from school and can't bear to be late to his swim practice, as much as he complains about going. At age eight, he announced that he wanted to be a chemist when he grows up. Teachers write effusive praise on his report cards. I swagger around when I visit his classroom.

Buzz isn't anxious, which I don't regret. But nor, at least to date, is he inspired, which deeply worries me, since I doubt he'd be satisfied by a run-of-the-mill life. I suspect that, like me, he's going to need to be driven by some urgent goal and swept up by his work, or flame out. And in our long forced march through the U.S. public school system, I've often felt that it was all I could do to prevent a flame-out before Buzz reached his teens.

Schools sabotage kids like Buzz all the time, in ways both subtle and dramatic. Todd Rose tells me he once visited a Massachusetts school district that was making hyperactive children wear *lead vests*. "They had a misconception that if you weighed the students down, it would stop them from moving, and thereby solve all the problems," he says. "But it just made things worse. The kids not only had backaches, but it made them look like idiots."

While Buzz escaped those vests, he has been weighed down in other ways. Teased and excluded in the schoolyard, he has been criticized in the classroom by a series of frustrated teachers who only rarely tried to understand him. *Try harder!* they've urged, making him feel even more like a loser. "He's *negligent!*" wailed his Spanish teacher, after giving him a detention for forgetting to bring his binder to class.

On one memorable afternoon, at the end of Buzz's seventh-grade year, I happened to pick him up from school just as all the other kids were out on the front lawn, signing each other's yearbooks. Buzz was alone, shoulders hunched as if he were trying to retract his head.

"Where's your yearbook?" I asked him, gnashing my teeth to think of the half dozen Post-its I'd used to remind myself to order and pay for it.

It turned out the librarian had withheld it, without calling me, because Buzz had a library book overdue. When we got home, I found the book underneath his bed and called the principal to complain, while the incident got me thinking how I might have reacted had Jack, for example, forbidden me from going to dinner with friends as a punishment for losing my keys—especially after making me sit still for several hours, berating me for chewing gum, and demanding that I raise my hand and ask permission, in front of everyone, every time I needed to use the bathroom.

Frankly, I'd be the opposite of inspired to behave well. Maybe I'd even invent a Tomás Mooger.

WITH PASSING YEARS and an escalating workload, Buzz's difficulties at school steadily worsened, leading to the emergency of his first year of middle school. The U.S. middle school system is a widely acknowledged failure; it has been dubbed the Bermuda Triangle of American education, where many kids get lost forever. Among seventeen industrialized nations ranked according to math achievement, U.S. fourth graders have come in at an already embarrassing ninth place—but they sink to twelfth place after completing middle school.

Is it really so puzzling? The U.S. middle school formula amounts to isolating hitherto cheerful elementary school kids who've morphed, as one teacher described it to me, into "hormones with legs," and sticking them at their desks for marathons of endurance, while steadily cutting back on previous allotments of recess, physical education, and lunch breaks.

The students suffer emotionally as well as academically, as is obvious from the perversely titled "Healthy Kids" surveys filled out yearly at Buzz's school. In his seventh-grade year, a full 20 percent of his peers described themselves as feeling so continuously sad or hopeless that they'd withdrawn from their normal activities—a hall-mark of clinical depression.

The boring routine of most classrooms is special torture for rest-less kids like Buzz, who once got a detention for dancing the ma-carena in his chair in Spanish class. One classic research study has shown that U.S. students spend as much as 50 percent of their class-time waiting for something to happen. With so much of the rest of the time devoted to prepping for tests, it's easy to see how those magic learning elements of excitement, relevance, and emotional connection can be dismissed as frills—by the staff, if not by the stu-dents.

At a particularly dispiriting meeting of that parent-teacher coun-cil that I finally quit attending, my eyes were glazing over as I strug-gled to follow the principal's droning reading of an outline promising to "develop and implement common formative assessments" to help raise math scores. Suddenly, one of the invited student representa-tives raised his hand and exclaimed: "You know, a lot of the kids are really bored! We don't see the point. Maybe it would be a good idea to make math more fun!" The principal and vice principal exchanged patient smiles. A couple of the teachers audibly sucked in their breath.

"Of course that's a good idea, Robert!" the principal said brightly, and then without another word returned to reading the proposition to "use the essential standards to guide district curriculum and as-sessment development . . ."

So could this have been any more ironic? Here young Robert was handing us a genuine learning opportunity, presented with the requi-site emotion and relevance, and—assuming Todd Rose and the neu-roscientists are right—delivering the key to raise those math scores. Couldn't we have cut the jargon even for a minute to talk about the ways teachers might connect lessons to things the kids care about? Alas, in the two and a half years I went to those meetings, we never did.

In his freewheeling class at Brigham and Women's Hospital, however, Rose keeps the challenge of engaging his class front and center. Sometimes, he tells me, he brings in a football playbook, the content of which can be as complicated as some physics problems, to demonstrate just how easily his "math-challenged" students can absorb it. Rose understands this problem from the inside: at the state college in Utah that he attended before he went to Harvard, he says he often spent more time figuring out why he should care about a subject than he did studying it. Once he did that, he says, "I was good to go."

"Will there ever come a day when parents can demand that schools engage their kids?" I ask him, as we sit on the school desks, at the end of his class. "Like, when we can say that boring them out of their minds amounts to child abuse?"

Rose laughs, but says, "You never know. Just remember, it used to be okay for teachers to hit them with sticks."

This has become a common sort of interchange for us, as Rose has generously expanded his role from wilderness guide to life coach. He tells me that Buzz and I just need to get through these few years, that these years are the hardest, and that I should be glad when I see evidence that Buzz's school hasn't yet crushed his spirit, specifically including the macarena incident. "Count your blessings," Rose says. "He's fighting back. He *could* just collapse and take the beating. A lot of kids do."

Even so, there are still so many times I get anxious as I wonder how Buzz will ever fit into a traditional classroom. At times like that, it helps to remember his exceptional year with Laura Graham.

Graham taught Buzz in fourth grade, during a year that easily could have turned into a total disaster. It was the year I first found out I was going to need brain surgery, and the same year Buzz was first diagnosed with ADD. Yet instead of floundering in school back then, he flourished. He got As and Bs, had only a few minor behavior problems, and danced and sang as the Artful Dodger in the school presentation of *Oliver!* He joined a baseball team and studied maps and atlases at night to compete in the geography bee. He actually liked going to school, which I know was largely due to Graham.

"She was never boring," Buzz has told me reverently.

Graham, in her forties, dressed and acted like someone half her age, with a long ponytail and a prankster's smile. She'd occasionally roll sideways down the grassy hill outside her classroom and once told me proudly how she'd taught some fifth graders about binary numbers with the Socratic method, "just to shake things up." What Buzz loved best were the tricks she played on the students she knew could handle some teasing, like getting the rest of the class to hide after one of them left to use the bathroom. Long before researchers publicized convincing evidence linking physical activity and academic performance, Graham began each day by having kids run laps and do calisthenics, and sometimes calling for a spontaneous "hokey pokey" when they got restless in the afternoon.

When I first told Graham about Buzz's diagnosis, she asked several questions that showed genuine interest, after which she eagerly collaborated with me to try to help him shine. She sent weekly reports home that graded him for progress on target behaviors that took special attention, such as doing his homework, making eye contact, and saying something kind about another person. We arranged that on the days he got high scores, I'd cook him bacon. Once, after he finally organized his desk, Graham took a photograph of him in front of it, drew big red hearts all over the picture, and sent it home, where we taped it to the refrigerator. Buzz "is very bright," she wrote on his report card, "and I eagerly await to see him reach his potential."

The vital importance of these sorts of relationships makes it all the more disheartening to consider the increasing odds against them, as U.S. classrooms grow more crowded and less manageable.

IT'S NO SECRET that American schools are in big trouble.

U.S. taxpayers, per capita, spend more on primary and secondary education than most other developed countries, in return for larger classes, lower test scores, and higher drop-out rates. There are a thousand points of blame for this failure, including teachers' low status and pay, the widely reviled state-mandated curricula, and, of course, America's increasingly distracted, stressed-out parents.

My own state, California, is in a special mess, ranking forty-seventh of fifty states in per-pupil education spending, even as a state budget crisis and a national recession threaten to make things much worse. As I write this, teachers in California are getting pink slips, class sizes are growing, and school administrators are spending most of their energy simply trying not to lose ground.

These pressures are cranking up a long-standing debate about whether public schools should even try to include rebellious, impulsive kids like Buzz—a concern I certainly understand. Unless those kids are getting what they need, a tall and rarely delivered order, they can suck all the oxygen out of a room. Even literally, like young Todd Rose and his handful of stink bombs.

Citing concerns about campus violence, many schools have been jettisoning young troublemakers with "zero tolerance" for behaviors that were often overlooked in the past. Yet researchers argue that the threat of violence has been overblown, while the harsh policies unfairly discriminate against clinically distracted kids who are bound to misbehave at least occasionally. The more tedious the school environment, the greater the odds are that such kids will be disruptive—a rule that finally inspired me to pull Buzz out of his problematic Spanish class after he got yet another detention, this time for raising his hand to protest the third consecutive showing of a cartoon video explaining how to use *"me gusta"* ("I like it") in a sentence. (He told me, and I believe him, that several kids stood up to applaud him as he left the room.)

The Harvard cognitive scientist David Rose—no relation to Todd—describes this sort of problem as more of a disabled school than a disabled child. "Schools are the perfect bad match for kids with attention deficit disorder," he tells me, when I reach him by phone, a few days after my trip to Boston. "We end up not only not educating them, we damage them."

Quite possibly, part of this damage is that many parents of even minimally disruptive children feel they have no alternative but to medicate kids who'd be just fine in a different environment. In other words, "if the schools were okay, we wouldn't need meds," as Susan

Smalley, an expert in the genetics of ADD at the University of California at Los Angeles, summed up to me in an interview.

While this remains a minority view, Smalley made a good case for it. In isolation, she told me, ADD is simply a human variability— part of what she calls "neurodiversity." It's only disabling in a badly matched environment. Like a six-foot-five guy getting out of a taxicab, instead of shooting hoops on a court. Or me being in charge of managing our family's finances, instead of finding new people to interview about new things. Smalley assured me that she didn't mean to suggest that I should stop giving Buzz his pill. Still, after talking with her and David Rose, I felt obligated to investigate whether there was anything I could do about what I was coming to see as my son's *environmental* disability.

IF YOU'RE LUCKY ENOUGH to live in San Diego and, on top of that, literally win a lottery, your child can enroll in one of eight charter schools in a widely acclaimed program known as High Tech High. The 2,500 student population roughly mirrors the local community, meaning there are just as many, and in some of the schools even more, kids with learning disabilities than in the public schools. The difference is that High Tech High's students all graduate, an achievement that has not been lost on parents. At this writing there are ten applications for every enrollee. Some families have even moved into the district from other parts of the state for the chance that a child might attend.

What's the secret? More than anything, as I find out, it's that the schools' administration genuinely recognizes the importance of engagement. Larry Rosenstock, the founding principal, tells me he tends to agree with Smalley's maybe-it's-not-so-radical-after-all view that we wouldn't need medication if the schools adapted to the kids, rather than vice versa. "Take a lot of these kids and put them in front of a massively complex, multiplayer, online role-playing game, and they'll figure it out without reading the instructions and, left to their own devices, do it ten hours a day," he said. "Isn't there something we can learn from this?"

High Tech High has a rigorous curriculum, but the rule rather than the exception is that students are out of their seats, involved in hands-on projects and teamwork. Teachers are encouraged to stray from the texts to make the work more interesting and meaningful. Science teacher Jay Vavra, for instance, has recruited students for a research project in which they isolate DNA from meat samples, as part of an effort to help an international conservation group devise better methods of identifying illegal bushmeat sold in African markets.

The charter school status allows High Tech High to avoid district-wide hiring constraints. Teachers are chosen in part based on classroom auditions and—*get this*—input from the students. They're paid more than other public school teachers, although they sacrifice job security. The contracts last only one year at a time, with performance continually under review. (Self-selected for exceptional idealism, most of the teachers make the cut.) Nor are the expectations limited to what happens in the classrooms. Teachers are also required to visit each of their students' families once a year and to advise small groups of students continuously throughout their time at the high school. Each student knows that there is at least one adult at the school who feels personally responsible for his or her success.

The first High Tech High school opened in 2000, as the fruit of efforts by local business executives who had united in their distress over the impact of public school failures on the future local workforce. The Bill and Melinda Gates Foundation donated funds to establish other campuses, but today all eight of the schools run on the same $6,900-per-pupil allocation that prevails in other public schools, thanks mostly to relatively lean overhead expenses.

The schools' special tactics for supporting all of their students are particularly helpful for kids with learning issues. Class sizes are smaller than the norm, and the teachers keep their focus on what the kids are learning rather than their learning style. As an example, premium quality note-taking assistance is available to all students, to avoid handicapping kids who haven't mastered that skill. At the start of the year, the teacher picks the best note-taker in the class, and pays that student $50 for the year to disseminate his or her records.

I first heard about High Tech High from psychologist Mark Katz, who works there on contract and who once organized a visit to the school by a group of psychiatrists specializing in attention deficit disorder. He called the tour "Beyond the Pill." The school, he says, is "a snapshot of what can happen if people let go of the rigidity that drives kids with attention issues crazy."

And so there *is* a public school heaven for quirky kids—at least for those lucky High Tech High students. Elsewhere, education pioneers are doing their best simply to improve hellish conditions. In Virginia, a team of researchers from James Madison University has organized a highly successful after-school program geared specifically for middle school students with attention deficit disorder. The program provides one-on-one mentoring sessions—similar to Buzz's private tutoring sessions with Blossom, minus the $65-an-hour fee— that help kids with common troubles such as note-taking, organizing backpacks, and getting their assignments written down. After ten years, the program has helped enrollees raise their grades, while reducing drop-out rates and behavior problems.

The U.S. public school system clearly still has far to go before parents of clinically distracted children no longer need to work so hard, spend so much, and maybe even make that hard decision to medicate. But the more I look, the more hopeful I feel that change is on the way. In Colorado, for instance, researchers have developed a two-year preschool curriculum called Tools of the Mind, with exercises demonstrated to improve the brain's "executive functions," including self-discipline and even working memory. Children learn to wait for their turns, for instance, with a "buddy reading" routine, in which one child reads aloud while another sits quietly, holding a picture of an ear. As word of this program's success has spread, more than 450 full and half-day classrooms, in six U.S. states, at this writing, have adopted it.

In an increasing number of U.S. schools, an even simpler intervention—aerobic exercise—has helped achieve dramatic improvements in the behavior of students with and without attention deficit disorder. These schools are bucking the national trend—today, barely 6 percent of U.S. high schools still offer daily physical education—but may eventually help reverse it, as they gather proof of success, with higher test scores and reduced disciplinary problems.

Todd Rose assures me that even more dramatic change for kids with learning disorders is on the way, via a concept known as Universal Design for Learning. The idea derives from the architectural notion that buildings should be accessible to all kinds of people—including people in wheelchairs and mothers with strollers—not only by means of costly add-ons, like ramps, but with more thoughtful, integral features like curb-cuts and automatic doors. Educators should take a similar approach, according to this theory, and be more intelligent about the ways they present material. Laptops might substitute for textbooks, for example, so that a dyslexic child might work on a computer that reads aloud to him, while an immigrant student might use a screen that lets him click on a phrase such as "George Washington" and see a pop-up explanation that Washington was the first U.S. president. Meanwhile, restless kids like Buzz wouldn't have so many chances to tune out, since the teachers would be wasting less time handing out papers or dealing with individual problems.

Initially designed for marginalized children, these tactics end up helping all students, the advocates say. In other words, kids like Buzz are the coal-miners' canaries. While they've been grimed by the school system's dysfunctions to date, they may just lead the way to reform.

ON A BRIGHT autumn afternoon, I'm sitting in my car, in the parking lot of a private school where Buzz has been "shadowing"—following a high school freshman around for the day. The school is determinedly college-prep, but with a reputation for "rescuing" children who've had trouble fitting into traditional classrooms.

There's no way we can afford it. The tuition—are you sitting down?—is $30,000 a year, comparable to other private high schools in the pricey San Francisco Bay Area. Jack and I would probably also end up having to drive Buzz on what would be his half-hour commute each way. On top of which, it's completely against our principles even to consider such an elitist escape route.

The whole idea is ridiculous, out of the question.

That said, I've been diligently filling out application forms, attending open houses, interviewing other parents, and praying that we can get financial aid.

Jack is still resisting. As a rule, he doesn't approve of spending money that we don't have. My father bought him the only two sports jackets he has owned as an adult—one of which he wore at our wedding.

I know that a good wife is supposed to cooperate and compromise. And I hate to push Jack to do something against his principles. On the other hand, there are no High Tech High schools in the Bay Area. At the high school Jack thinks Buzz should attend, just five blocks from our house, there are as many as thirty kids in a class, and, by the way, the district has one of the nation's highest rates of binge drinking.

In contrast, the private school we're considering has just eight kids to a teacher, and the teachers—I've watched them—are energized. It looks like a place that might just understand Buzz, and I can tell, as he runs out the front door now to meet me, that he agrees. He's grinning exuberantly, holding up a wooden plank he made with a laser in an art class, on which he has inscribed the word "COW-BOYS," with two large stars, for his favorite football team.

"This place is GREAT!" he says. *When did I last hear him talk about school, or anything, for that matter, with this sort of enthusiasm?*

"Let's just see if he gets in, before you freak out," I tell Jack when Buzz and I get home. As for me, I'm already thinking that maybe we won't retire as early as we had planned, or ever. Or maybe we can sell something. (*A kidney?*) Because seemingly overnight, following this shadowing visit, Buzz for the first time in several years is talking and acting as if he cares about school.

Within the week, he has finished a draft of his application essay, which asks him to describe someone who has influenced him. He chooses to describe his meeting with Todd Rose, telling all about Rose's high school failure, and how he bounced back, and how happy he looked teaching the class at the hospital. "He made a difference to me because I'd thought that if you get below a 3.0 grade point average, you couldn't excel in life," Buzz writes. "Todd gave me the hope, though, and now I know that even if I mess up a little, I can still get myself out of the hole and excel just like he did."

I think back to that morning in Boston, when I'd assumed Buzz hadn't been paying attention. Just shows how much I know.

CHAPTER 7

ADD-VOCACY

The Strength in Numbers

I felt it shelter to speak to you.

EMILY DICKINSON

BUZZ AND I ARE SITTING TOGETHER IN THE BACK ROW OF A packed conference room at the Anaheim, California, convention center. People have begun to introduce themselves, just as if we're at a meeting of Alcoholics Anonymous:

"I'm Shirley. I'm a nurse from Toronto, Canada, and I have attention deficit disorder."

"I'm Maria from New Jersey. I have three kids and a husband with attention deficit disorder."

"I'm Gloria, and I have a three-year-old with attention deficit disorder and oppositional defiant disorder."

"I'm Robert. I have a son who says he doesn't have attention deficit disorder."

I look around. There are about sixty people here, most of them thoroughly fried-looking women of about my age, plus two men who may be fathers, a smattering of doctors and therapists, and three fidgeting young men, the youngest of which is Buzz. All of us are first-time attendees at the twentieth annual international conference of CHADD: Children and Adults with Attention-Deficit/

Hyperactivity Disorder, the leading U.S. support group for the seriously distracted.

This introductory workshop is designed to help us first-timers feel more at ease amid more than one thousand other attendees at the four-day gathering. That's standard operating procedure, not only for CHADD, but for the bevy of other American mental-health advocacy groups, focused on linking people together in the intimate way that only a shared mental disorder can do. In the past couple of decades, more than a dozen such organizations have sprung up in the United States and, most recently, even in countries as new to the self-help concept as Saudi Arabia. By uniting people (and their families) with maladies including ADD, autism, Tourette's syndrome, and schizophrenia, these groups have helped conquer stigma and fulfill a deep yearning for shared experience and information.

It's a major public service that also has a dark side. Several of these groups, including CHADD, depend heavily on donations and advertising funds from big drug companies, which in CHADD's case supplied nearly one-third of its FY 2008 revenues of $4.2 million. The alliance is nothing if not pragmatic, given the shared goal of spreading the word that mental illness is genuine, serious, and often treatable with prescription medications. Yet as public trust in the drug firms has declined, in the wake of recalls of unsafe medications and congressional investigations questioning lavish payments to researchers, the advocacy groups' public image has suffered by association.

CHADD's ties with Big Pharma are conspicuous at the Anaheim meeting. As I look around the room, it strikes me that I and my fellow first-time conference-goers look like walking sandwich-board ads for stimulant medications, with our big red tote bags, emblazoned with the logo for Shire, which makes the amphetamine Adderall, and, around our necks, the red-and-white nametag ribbons that say, "McNeil Pediatrics," the manufacturer of Concerta.

But now Buzz jolts me out of my reverie, joyfully kicking my ankle to make sure I heard the woman who has just told the group: "I have ADD worse than my son does."

Soon it will be his turn to speak.

Anne Teeter Ellison (no relation to me), the departing president of CHADD, presides over the meeting. She's statuesque, with auburn, shoulder-length hair, a look of bristly impatience, and a lapel sticker that reads "AD/HD IS REAL." As she nods at each new introduction, it hits me—only now—that in all the talks that Buzz and I have had this year, I've never once heard him mention the disorder by name.

Until this moment, I haven't ever weighed the consequences of my son's publicly assuming this diagnostic label. *Is it really a good idea for Buzz to talk about himself this way?* "Attention *deficit* disorder." It's so *pessimistic*. On the other hand, might claiming his part in this eccentric community make him feel less alone? Give him a sense of defiant pride, of overcoming obstacles?

I put my arm around Buzz's shoulders and whisper, "You don't have to say anything if you don't want to!"

Buzz whispers back: "I'm going to say my *brother* has it!"

But then it's his turn, and he just flashes a smile and says, "I'm Buzz, and I've got attention deficit disorder."

Relief sweeps over me. He makes it sound like no big deal.

"I'm Kathy," I say. "I'm Buzz's mom, and I've got it, too."

IT WAS ONLY two days ago that I decided to bring Buzz along on this trip. I'd been dreaming of one of those rare hotel-room respites where time flows without frantic interruptions and I get to interview people over lunch and watch movies in bed at night, by myself, and don't even have to think about how much Xbox the kids are playing in my absence.

Besides, I figured, bringing Buzz would be impractical for reasons beyond the cost. What with his recent bar mitzvah preparations, plus all the neurofeedback sessions, he'd fallen way behind in his schoolwork. So when he asked if he could join me, I decided to be strategic. Crafty. I didn't have to say no; I could just set the bar impossibly high.

"Sure!" I said, stifling a smile. "Just as long as you finish all your overdue homework! I'll give you a day."

Buzz nodded his head, like a quarterback in a huddle, sat down at the computer, and within ninety minutes had caught himself up.

Well, maybe it's not such a bad idea, I thought, even as I struggled to appease Max, who was not only enraged that I was taking yet another trip without him, but somehow had figured out how close we'd be to Disneyland.

"Buzz gets to go everywhere, just because he has problems!" Max protested.

"Look, I understand why it seems that way to you, and I'd really like to spend some special time with you when we get back," I said. "Where would you like to go?"

"Some place Buzz hasn't been!"

I calmed him down as best I could, assuring him we'd be staying at a boring hotel, and that we wouldn't be doing anything but work, and I'm keeping that promise, despite how Buzz began lobbying, the minute our plane landed, to skip the meetings and go ride the Matterhorn. Nope, we're sticking to our dutiful agenda, as I encourage him to try to appreciate the amusement-park aura of the meeting itself, attracting the clinically distracted and those who study us from as far away as Italy, Uruguay, and the Netherlands.

There are workshops teaching everything from the importance of aerobic exercise, to what to do about bullying, to how to negotiate public schools and health insurance, to approaches to niche dilemmas for people with ADD who are also gays and lesbians, single parents, women and girls, and—I kid you not—Argentine preschoolers. There's an elaborate lunch buffet and free gifts, including boxes of tissues and alarm clocks branded with the names of stimulant meds. An auditorium is packed with booths hawking a startling array of products and services tailored to the clinically distracted: individualized coaching, summer camps, brain-training software, fish oil, little watchbands that vibrate to remind you to take your medication, and snack bars with omega-3 supplements.

Our schedules list talks by Bruce Jenner, the 1976 Olympic decathlon champion who says he struggled with childhood "attention issues" and dyslexia, and Jay Giedd, chief of the brain-imaging unit at the National Institute of Mental Health. There are sessions on genetic research, meditation, diet, neurofeedback, social skills, and "Healthy Helicopter Parenting." It's potentially overwhelming, as Teeter Ellison acknowledges at the newcomers' orientation.

"Look at your schedules and make a plan," she advises us. "Decide the best use of your time, and then, if you see something new out there, just file it away. Don't let yourself get distracted by the new."

TEETER ELLISON'S informed empathy epitomizes the sunny side of CHADD, which has helped spur an evolution in understanding and compassion for a disorder so widely still seen as a character flaw. The group is an information powerhouse, with its U.S. government–sponsored, bilingual data bank, its annual conventions, its Web site, and its glossy magazine, annually distributed to forty thousand U.S. doctors' offices.

CHADD is also an accomplished lobbyist. From its headquarters in Landover, Maryland, just outside Washington, D.C., the organization has joined several similar mental health advocacy groups in obtaining research funds and laws protecting clinically distracted folk in schools and in the workplace. A major triumph came in 2008, with the passage of a mental health parity bill—a long-awaited big step forward in getting insurance firms to help share the burden of expensive mental health care for millions of policyholders.

Where I suspect CHADD has made just as deep a difference, however, is in its grassroots support of local groups of parents who help one another cope, week to week. In its twenty-two years of existence, CHADD has trained and certified 261 parents to be volunteer leaders of local community support groups.

I sit in on a "Parent-to-Parent" (or P2P) training session at the convention, while Buzz, who got restless during the newcomers' workshop, takes a break to watch part of a basketball game on TV in our room upstairs. There are about forty other women at the training session, plus three men (one of whom leaves early). We sit at school desks with hefty, hard-bound manuals: our texts for a curriculum that stretches over fourteen hours.

I've been to a CHADD support group a couple of times back home, so I'm already familiar with the basic approach. Most of the focus is where it's most desperately needed: on practical advice about how to keep the love alive when you're annoyed, frustrated, over-taxed, and exhausted.

"We talk about relationships in every single session," Mary Durheim, CHADD's educational consultant, informs the prospective volunteer leaders. "Relationships are everything." What remains unspoken, yet which every parent in the room with an extremely difficult child re-mains terribly aware of, is that even the supposedly sacred ties be-tween mothers and children aren't invulnerable. That sometimes love doesn't come naturally, and sometimes it can even disappear.

Durheim and the other two group leaders—self-assured, battle-scarred moms—proceed with the shared understanding that some-times love takes a lot of work, combined with some Herculean understanding. They keep reminding us of the biological origins of ADD, meaning that much of our children's "bad" behavior really can't be helped. ("Think of the meltdowns as "behavioral seizures," we're told.) They urge us to keep in mind that our kids may be fight-ing battles at school every day, with teachers and peers, that contrib-ute to making them angry and impossible at home.

"The most debilitating effect of ADD is loss of self-esteem," says Durheim. "So we must see the individual as *in* trouble, not as the *cause* of trouble."

Next comes a rapid-fire discussion of tips to help make home life easier. Keep a picture of your child as a baby on the refrigerator—"to remind yourself *this is your baby!*" Dole out praise as much as possi-ble, and give only "positive" instructions—e.g., "Keep your hands to yourself!" instead of "Don't hit your brother!"

"You want to teach parents to see the small changes," another one of the moms, Beth Kaplanek, advises her class. "Are their children getting up out of bed in the morning with three reminders, not six? Right!" She snaps her fingers for emphasis. "You got it!"

Mixed in with all the empathy on view at the P2P meeting is a heavy dose of tough love. Durheim sternly addresses the risks of credit cards—"*Never* give 'em to these kids!"—and reports that there's a new way of putting GPS on a cell phone without your son or daughter knowing. Next up comes the topic of drug screens. Durheim is not only in favor of periodic urine samples as a check on teenagers' veracity, but urges parents to take precautions against attempted fraud. "I hate to say this," she says. "But you gotta stand there and watch them do it."

I take a moment to gaze around the room, at all these earnest, worried moms. It's been nearly a half century since the dawn of the supposed feminist revolution, yet all that time has hardly made a dent in the bottom-line difference between mothers and fathers, the difference that makes all the difference, which is that *mothers worry more*. That right there is the three-word explanation for why Jack has felt free to spend hours every evening watching baseball games and doing his crossword puzzles, while I've been anguishing over all those parenting books. And why he's not here with me now, taking notes on the P2P meeting and nervously plotting our strategy for when Buzz starts driving, four years from now.

There are times, like right now, when I start worrying about how much I've been worrying, and wonder if Jack's carefree style might actually be better for Buzz. After all, Jack turned out okay, after being raised mostly by his own dad, a tough World War II vet who managed movie theaters by night and stayed home by day with his three kids while Jack's mother played violin as a member of the Los Angeles Philharmonic. Jack has told me how, when he was still an infant, his father took him out for ribs at the end of his shift late one night. When a female diner grimaced at the baby with his face smeared with barbeque sauce, Jack's father shot back, "Lady, does he look like he's suffering?"

In Rio, when Jack and I first started clashing over our parenting styles, we visited a marriage counselor—a man—who suggested to me that when I see Jack with his feet up, watching TV, I should put my feet up, too. And I could almost imagine doing that, if I also knew that Jack would be the one to get up to humbly answer the phone the next time Buzz's teacher called to complain. Or check Buzz's agenda to see if he even wrote down his homework. Or make sure his gym clothes are washed, even though he refuses to suit up for PE.

WALKING BACK to the room to get Buzz after the Parent-to-Parent training, I'm actually quite proud of myself for the way I've already been incorporating many of the basic principles into my parenting, what with my bombing-with-love campaign over the past several weeks. And I daresay I've already seen some results. Buzz has all but stopped haranguing me to buy him outrageous or unaffordable gifts. And he seems to be picking fights less often. Still, he's clearly got the same amount of mental energy, which he uses these days to pepper me with questions. Not the Max kind of questions, which test my knowledge, but thornier issues of personal taste and ethics, to which he needs answers *right now*.

"What would you rather eat, sirloin steak or salmon?" he asked a few days ago, as I was kneeling to peer under a dresser, searching for another lost earring.

"I dunno, it depends on how I'm feeling! Is the steak grass-fed? Is the salmon wild?"

"You don't know, but you have to choose!"

A minute later, it was: "Mom, you have to choose. Either George Bush gets reelected, or Max loses a tiny bit of his earlobe!"

"I'm not going to make that kind of choice! Take *my* earlobe!"

In another sign of progress, Buzz's behavior in public has become a lot more civilized, so much so that I've dared to invite him along today to an important interview. I've set up a lunch meeting with Blake Taylor, the young author of a new book about his own experiences with attention deficit disorder (*ADHD & Me*), and his mother, Nadine Taylor-Barnes. Blake, who was diagnosed as a child, is now taking premed classes at the University of California at Berkeley. He also speaks French, plays classical piano, and does volunteer work caring for abandoned greyhound dogs.

Buzz is wearing his blue Terrell Owens jersey and oversized white LA Dodgers cap. We get to the hotel restaurant a few minutes late, because he somehow lost the cap within the confines of our small hotel room, and refused to leave until he found it, on the floor, under a heap of his clothes.

Blake is waiting alone at a table. I recognize his blond crew cut from the book-jacket picture, and notice a sleepy cast to his eyes, an expression he shares with Buzz.

Nadine still hasn't come down from their room.

"She's late again," Blake says. "Let's just order."

The waiter is bringing out an appetizer plate of quesadillas as Nadine rushes in, apologizing. A former global communications manager for IBM, she's not only smart and accomplished, but strikingly pretty: slender, with long blond hair. I notice a wearily anxious look in her eyes, an expression she shares with me.

Five minutes into the quesadillas, she and Blake are arguing. She's trying to convince him to go up to their room and get his laptop so he can register online for a course he needs before it fills up. He wants her off his case.

"*Jesus,* Mims!" he finally shouts. "*I don't need to do it right now!*"

This prompts another of Buzz's kicks under the table. Buzz calls me something similar: "Meem," which he says he got from the TV cartoon *South Park*.

"Stop *kicking* me!" I hiss at my son. He shows no sign of hearing, grinning away in his hope of more fireworks.

But Blake, having said his piece and finished his burger, now agrees to go up to the room. And even though Buzz stays at the table—tucking into the banana split he managed to order while I was distracted talking to Nadine—I launch into the sensitive questions that really led me to ask for this lunch. Impressed as I am by Blake, I'm more eager to know how Nadine pulled this off, managing to raise such an accomplished (if still rather exasperating) son, despite the disorder that devastates so many lives.

Nadine smiles her warm smile and patiently tells me how her marriage suffered—she's now divorced—and she gave up her high-powered job along the road leading to Blake's triumphs. "I'm a serious feminist," she assures me, before explaining how she recognized she had to make a choice between her children and her career after the day she caught five-year-old Blake hiding in the corporate limousine that had come to take her to the airport for another business trip. "I was getting blamed big-time," Nadine says. "My mom said, 'You're working too much—that's why he's acting up.'"

Ah, CHADD. I come for the workshops; I stay for the schadenfreude. . . .

Over the next several years, Blake kept Nadine on her toes, figuring out how to open "child-safe" Tylenol bottles as a tot, lighting the dining room tablecloth on fire, and setting off alarms in museums. She poured her energy into finding the right therapists and coaches, and tutoring her son herself, every day after school, and getting Blake on the right meds and into a supportive private school. She also forced him—at least initially, despite his angry objections—into a rigorous exercise routine. "I'd pick him up at his train home from school and drive him, kicking and screaming, right to the gym, where a trainer would be waiting," she tells me.

I nod, rapt. Nadine should have been leading the Parent-to-Parent training. She has it *down*.

There's no time for coffee, since the workshops are starting again, and there's a talk on the benefits of aerobic exercise I think Buzz might like. We say our good-byes, and on the way up the escalator together, I restrain my urge to pester him about what he thought of Blake, much less his awesomely devoted mother. As for me, I'm both dazzled and exhausted. *There is always so much more you can do. . . .*

I DID SOME research into CHADD's origins in the weeks before the Anaheim conference, and discovered that it began in the town of Plantation, Florida, as the shared vision of a psychologist, a speech therapist, and a mother, Fran Gilman, whose son the two professionals were

treating. The boy, as Gilman told me in a telephone interview, had
been kicked out of half a dozen preschools for disruptive behavior before his fifth birthday. That was 1987, and few parents, teachers, or
even many doctors knew much of substance about attention deficit
disorder. Instead, kids often got other, usually much crueler labels,
such as "retards," "pests," and "juvenile delinquents." And their parents
shouldered much of the blame.

"The isolation and the stigma were horrible, horrible," Gilman
told me, with seemingly fresh sadness. "And the unsolicited advice
was copious. But no one ever said anything like 'Jeez, Fran, you look
tired.'"

This was 1987, still seven years before the media frenzy over attention deficit disorder, and even longer before people could attempt
to quench their thirst for information on the Internet. Together with
Harvey Parker, the psychologist, and Carol Lerner, the speech therapist, Gilman was eager to see if other parents felt the same need as
she did for information and support. "Not only could we maybe find
a common thread in connecting, but we could help each other and
give support, like, okay, I found something that works in this situation, what about you?" Gilman told me.

They took out local ads and handed out fliers. Fifty eager parents
showed up at their first meeting. For the next meeting, they rented a
room at the Holiday Inn, but were still surprised when some 150
people turned up. Parents, mostly mothers, "just came out of the
woodwork," as Lerner recalled. By the third meeting, the trio had
decided to form a nonprofit organization, originally called Children
with Attention Deficit Disorders.

Soon, the new group was getting calls from other counties, and
before the year had ended, Florida had half a dozen chapters. Within
five years, several hundred chapters were active throughout the United
States, claiming some thirty-one thousand members.

These pre-Web years were the heyday of patient advocacy groups,
which had a lock on the most up-to-date information. The Autism
Society of America had been established in 1965, followed by the
National Tourette Syndrome Association, in 1972, and NAMI, the

National Alliance on Mental Illness, in 1979. As time went on, most
of these groups, including CHADD, established offices in the Washington, D.C., area, all the better to represent the legislative interests
of their members. CHADD was barely four years old and still in
Florida, however, when it achieved its first major political victory.
The organization's leaders convinced U.S. Department of Education
officials to stipulate to state education agencies that children diagnosed with ADD should be included in federal antidiscrimination
and special education laws. This watershed naturally led to a lot
more interest by parents in getting their children diagnosed, which
would justify more support at school. As critics point out, it also
ended up significantly expanding the market for pharmaceutical
stimulants.

In time, CHADD became the go-to place for media seeking responses to skeptics' questions about the validity of the ADD diagnosis and the use of stimulants to treat it. CHADD officials have
publicly taken on critics, including the Scientologist actor Tom Cruise,
who called Ritalin a "street drug" on NBC-TV, and the *New York
Times*' Maureen Dowd, for a column about "rampant" Ritalin abuse,
which mockingly suggested that a "fidgety" George Bush, then president, suffered from ADD.

"Almost on a day-to-day basis, we're bombarded with media mis-
conceptions coming out of the antipsychiatric movement that thinks
mental illness is a fraud," Teeter Ellison complained at the Anaheim
conference. In response, the group's leaders patiently cite each new
research finding suggesting physical differences in the brains of clinically distracted subjects, trusting that the weight of scientific data
may one day quell one of the fiercest debates in medical history. The
critics continue their attacks nonetheless, brushing aside CHADD's
protests as tainted by financial self-interest. In 2000, CHADD was
even named as a codefendant, along with drug manufacturers and
the American Psychiatric Association, in three civil suits charging a
conspiracy to boost sales of Ritalin.

"We saw CHADD as the marketing arm of the pharmaceutical
industry," plaintiff attorney Andy Waters told me. The lawyers never

managed to prove that case—the suits were dismissed within three years—but the credibility problems have lingered. Todd Rose canceled his CHADD membership after attending a 2003 convention where the drugmakers' blatant influence gave him an "icky, dirty feeling."

Rose is no foe of medication: he tells me he has taken stimulants nearly every day for the past decade. "But the problem is, you cannot argue against your economic interests," he says. "It just doesn't work. I love so much of what CHADD does, particularly the parent training. But the bottom line is it's just too easy a vehicle for drug companies."

IT WAS HARVEY PARKER, the psychologist cofounder of CHADD, who first opened the door to Big Pharma.

Just a few months after the group was established, he wrote to Ciba-Geigy, then the manufacturer of Ritalin, to ask for a donation. "They sent a check—for $500, or $1,000," he told me in a telephone interview. "It was a long time ago. I don't even remember what we used it for."

Some of the group's members objected even then to taking money from the drug firms, Parker acknowledged, adding, "There was always concern. We didn't want to give the impression we were being dictated to, which is why we set limits on how much we'd accept."

The guideline today is that no more than 30 percent of non-advertising revenue may come from pharmaceutical firms. It's actually not that tight a limit, especially considering that the same firms purchased $466,104 worth of ads in FY 2008. Most of the rest of the budget comes from members' dues, a federal government grant, and admission revenues from the yearly convention. Yet the trend in recent years has been for membership—and dues—to decline, while drug-manufacturer support has increased.

By the spring of 2009, the number of dues-paying members had fallen to just twelve thousand, according to CHADD spokesman Bryan Goodman. He attributed most of that drop to the rise of the Internet, with its more convenient, "virtual" support groups.

My guess is that CHADD's falling membership numbers haven't

chased away the drug firms for the simple reason that the firms have few better options these days to reach their target audience. And may I just add, what a wonderful target we are!

When you stop and think about it, clinically distracted people are a market made in heaven. Our numbers alone are enticing: an estimated 9 million American adults, and at minimum 4.5 million children—all of us, by definition, impulsive and novelty-seeking as well as often anxious and desperate. One-click shopping was *invented* with people like us in mind.

Over the past several decades, American drug firms have enjoyed exceptional freedom in courting consumers, although so great is the mounting public cynicism that even some clinically uninhibited people are no longer so easily seduced by mere ads. A U.S. survey in 2005 found that only 18 percent of consumers—compared to nearly twice that rate just eight years earlier—said they thought pharmaceutical ads could be trusted "most of the time."

This trend has made Big Pharma all the more eager to find warm and fuzzy trappings for its come-ons. So naturally they've zeroed in on family-friendly support groups, such as CHADD, NAMI, and another ADD group called the Attention Deficit Disorder Association. More recently, they've also started to colonize cyberspace, with McNeil Pediatrics, the manufacturer of Concerta, launching a Facebook page for "ADHD Moms" in 2008.

McNeil's PR department came up with this idea after its market research revealed that mothers of clinically distracted children were feeling isolated and stigmatized and were wandering Internet social networking sites by night. "We thought we could put the information in their comfort zone," McNeil spokeswoman Trish Geoghegan proudly told me, in a phone interview.

The page, unsurprisingly, is especially comforting in regards to the hard decision to treat children's clinical distraction with stimulants. Handpicked testimonials from some of the more than eight thousand "fans," displayed on the page, have encouraged readers not only not to feel ashamed, but also to expect some awesome outcomes: sweeter, quieter kids, even "more focused" dancing.

The Facebook page is considered "unbranded" advertising. Because it doesn't mention Concerta by name, it's not required to list the drug's possible side effects, such as stunted growth, increased blood pressure, tics, and psychosis. What's more, the "average moms" and paid consultants are free to make artfully misleading claims. I listen to a podcast conversation in which an "average mom" is supposedly asking advice from a pediatrician—a paid McNeil consultant—about whether to take her son off his meds on weekends or during vacations. Such "drug holidays" are recommended by leading attention deficit experts, who say parents periodically should check to see if children no longer need their medication, and also give them a chance to catch up in height. McNeil's pediatrician is adamant, however, in encouraging the "average mom" to keep her child on stimulants, day in and day out. It's important for "the family interaction," the drug consultant says, adding that keeping her own child on meds allowed the family to go to Disneyland in an RV.

Groups like CHADD, which depend on the drug firms, may find themselves tarnished by association with such sneaky tactics. Which would be a real shame, undermining the truly worthwhile information and solace they might otherwise provide.

CHADD SPOKESMAN Bryan Goodman assures me that Big Pharma funding has never swayed the group's agenda. CHADD prides itself on taking a "multimodal" approach to ADD, he says, in which medication, behavioral therapy, and even some alternative treatments can all play important parts. Indeed, during my year of paying attention to attention, CHADD went on record to support federal research into neurofeedback—a particularly controversial approach—for clinical distraction.

At the same time, however, CHADD is increasingly reaching out to other countries where both ADD awareness and stimulant sales are growing rapidly. The Anaheim convention features both an "International Forum" and an "Iberoamerican Forum," packed mostly with medical professionals, flocking in from Germany, Switzerland,

Israel, Spain, and elsewhere. Many of them belong to new, CHADD-style support groups that have sprouted up in other countries over the past decade. Some have had their trips paid for by pharmaceutical firms, whose interest in this trend is obvious.

While the United States still represents more than 80 percent of global market share for ADD drugs, at this writing the market in developing nations is growing annually by double-digit figures. My concern on first hearing of this trend is tempered by a brief conversation I have at the CHADD meeting with a youthful pediatric neurologist named Soad Al Yamani, who treats children at the King Faisal Hospital in Riyadh. Al Yamani also runs Saudi Arabia's only ADD support group, an organization that, she tells me, grew to six thousand people within just two years after she founded it in 2004. "We're overwhelmed," she says, wincing. "My cell phone never stops because they've finally found someone who helps." Most clinically distracted Saudi children are never diagnosed, she explains, while most families reject the use of medication for mental disorders, even including epilepsy.

Al Yamani doesn't want to talk about America's "Ritalin Wars"—they're a luxury she can't afford. She tells me, instead, about her own, clinically distracted brother—a "brilliant" young unemployed drug addict—and describes how often she sees children with ADD at her clinic who've been physically abused by their families. "Parents in your country have gone through a lot of growth," she says wistfully.

I'm still thinking about Al Yamani as Buzz and I board the plane to fly back to San Francisco. I'm sure she was right to persuade me to recognize just how far Americans have come, so recently, in understanding mental disorders, as much as we're still drowning in data and confused by endless controversies. Yet I also know that the self-awareness that Buzz has been acquiring—even just on this trip with me—is a double-edged sword. There's that uncertainty about what it all means: the label of being disordered, the danger that he'll use his "disability" as an excuse. Even so, groups like CHADD offer kids like Buzz a powerful connection—not only a personal entry point with state-of-the-art research that may help him, increasingly, as he grows up, but also a tie to this eccentric but heartfelt community of fellow scatterbrains: with Todd Rose, and Blake Taylor, and lots of Brazilians and Costa Ricans and Saudis, and me.

The plane starts to move down the runway. I've been on hundreds of flights, in my years as a wandering journalist—on jets, military transport planes, helicopters, and once, a battered Cessna that made an unforgettable emergency landing in Brazil's northeastern desert after the radio gave out. I still get nervous during takeoffs and landings. *Takeoffs and landings are the most perilous moments of any flight.*

I've mentioned this to Buzz, but I'm still surprised and touched when he reaches over to hold my hand. I smile and kiss his forehead.

"So, what'd you think of all that, back there?" I ask, as we tilt up into the sky.

Buzz smiles back. As usual, he is a young man of few words.

"I've got the GOOD kind of ADD," he murmurs. "And YOU'VE got the boring kind!"

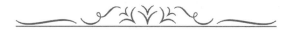

IS IT
CURABLE?

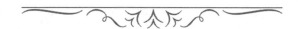

CHAPTER 8

WIRED

Braving the New World of Neurofeedback

Almost any problem will improve if you pay attention to it.

GENE ARNOLD, MD

Ohio State University professor emeritus,
and principal investigator of the first
federally sponsored study of neurofeedback

BUZZ LEANS BACK INTO A PADDED BLUE ARMCHAIR IN A DIMLY lit room.

Stretched over his head is a yellow rubber cap studded with nineteen gold, spoon-shaped electrodes: tiny microphones picking up the whisper of the electrical activity inside his skull. Colored wires lead from the cap to a small black box, which processes the information and feeds it into a laptop computer.

Standing just behind my son, I peer over his shoulder at the computer monitor. An undulating needle is producing an electroencephalogram, an EEG, drawing waves like you'd see on a seismograph. In this case, however, the little quakes represent my son's ever-changing mental states. The EEG is our first step in exploring a time-consuming, costly, and extremely controversial yet increasingly widespread, high-tech therapy called neurofeedback—biofeedback for the brain. Our long-term goal is for Buzz to learn how to be more calm and focused, by responding to a computer's repeated prompts to change his brain's habitual reactions.

Buzz has agreed to return to this office in San Rafael, California, for as many as forty half-hour sessions. I've enticed him with promises of dim sum and cash, but he also seems on board with the general plan. In recent decades, biofeedback has been an increasingly popular, computer-based approach to reducing the physical symptoms of stress—training people to slow down their own heart rates, for instance, with encouraging noises and visual displays. And more recently, the idea that we can change our very brains—the way we think and feel—in the same way, has been gaining traction. In each of these appointments, Buzz essentially will be playing video games with his brain instead of his thumbs. As long as he generates the desired mental state—staying calm, but alert—a Pac-Man will scoot around a maze, puzzle pieces will fall into place, or a racing car will speed ahead, and Buzz, presumably, will be encouraged to keep it up. "Your brain is like a puppy dog that likes to be rewarded," explains our practitioner, Cynthia Kerson.

I'm encouraged to imagine Buzz's brain still funny and sharp but, finally, house-trained. He seems to like Kerson, and is already being unusually cooperative, smiling and readily following directions. As I look back and forth from his face to the monitor, I feel a surge of affection that brings to mind the memory of my first sonogram. The clinic technician rolled a slippery sensor over my belly to reveal Buzz's embryonic outline, to the underwater sound of his beating heart. *And now, right there on that monitor, it's as if I can see inside his brain. . . .*

"DON'T TOUCH THAT CHAIR!"

Kerson's voice makes me jump. Lost in my reverie, I hadn't realized I'd rested an elbow just above Buzz's head, possibly disturbing the wires.

Kerson is a native New Yorker with straight, ash-brown hair, large gray eyes, and an edgy intelligence. At thirty-six, while running a multinational button-selling business, she was diagnosed with Graves' disease, an immune disorder that sent her thyroid into overdrive, making her thin and restless. She took a chance on the fringy new biofeedback for the brain, and promptly became one of the industry's most dedicated advocates. Neurofeedback "saved my life," Kerson tells me. She sold her button business, trained as a practitioner, and eventually became executive director of a membership group, the International Society for Neurofeedback and Research.

I'm going to get my own EEG after Kerson finishes this one for Buzz. She'll later compare our patterns with a database of so-called "normal" brains to produce a "brain map," otherwise known as a quantitative EEG, or QEEG. Each map costs $750, and that's just for starters. If we proceed, as planned, with forty half-hour sessions for each of us, the bill will come to $6,800. It's the most expensive therapy I've yet considered, not to mention all the time I'll have to take off from work, and it will eat up a considerable part of my book advance.

But frankly, I'm psyched. Neurofeedback is the new, new thing for attention deficit disorder—and anxiety, oppositional behavior, depression, bipolar disorder, autism, closed head injuries, migraines, seizures, premenstrual tension, chronic fatigue syndrome, alcoholism, smoking, and pretty much you name it in the realm of brain-based suffering, which basically amounts to *all* suffering. At this writing, some ten thousand children throughout the world are undergoing this therapy, as Kerson estimates. More than half of them are U.S. children with attention issues.

Increasing numbers of parents are plunking down the money, their hopes raised by intriguing preliminary research and abundant testimonials from former patients and practitioners. "Part of the problem with this field is that the stories are so amazing that nobody believes them. I'm trying not to sound like a wild man," says Laurence Hirshberg, a Brown University assistant professor in clinical psychiatry who also runs a large neurofeedback clinic.

The field, to be sure, has some equally impassioned and highly credentialed critics, who charge that researchers have yet to produce any "gold-standard" peer-reviewed studies conclusively proving that it works. The critics have also called attention to flaws in some of the optimistic preliminary reports—from the way research subjects were selected, to how results were compared among groups—and some simply dismiss the whole practice as, at best, a placebo: an expensive, time-consuming sugar pill. The prominent ADD researcher

William Pelham has included neurofeedback on a list he likes to recite of common but ineffective interventions—along with "horse therapy" and "duct tape."

The criticisms give me pause, but not for long. Neurofeedback makes sense to me, given all that scientists have learned over the past couple decades about the brain's ability to change itself—a concept known as "plasticity." What's more, I've got prestigious company in my willingness to test it out. Just this year, on the strength of a critical mass of studies with positive results, the U.S. National Institutes of Health has embarked on the first government-backed study of whether neurofeedback can help alleviate the symptoms of clinical distraction. The project's leader, Ohio State professor emeritus Gene Arnold, a nationally respected child psychiatry researcher, says the pilot project should yield results sometime in 2011, potentially leading to a larger trial. "Based on previous reports, we're expecting attention to improve, and if the children have hyperactive-impulsive behavior, we think that will get better, too," he tells me, in a phone interview, adding, "The theory is that it will have a permanent effect."

THE WEEK AFTER Buzz and I have our brains mapped, I return to Kerson's office with Jack on a Monday morning when Jack is off work and Buzz is in school. She hands over two illustrated reports packed with statistical information that sails right over our heads. I've ordered a few books on neurofeedback, but they haven't yet arrived, and I suppose it's not fair to expect Kerson to give me a class in the technique during what's supposed to be a brief appointment.

I ask a couple questions anyway, but then close my notebook with a sigh. Jack just sits and nods, his eyes glassy. He's much more skeptical about all this than I am, which is only one of the reasons I haven't yet gotten around to telling him how much it'll cost.

Over the next few weeks, I'll gradually get more of a handle on what we're getting into, as we move from a chemical to an electrical model of the glitch I appear to share with Buzz. Here's the basic narrative: Throughout the day and night, our hundred billion or so neurons, or brain cells, generate a constant storm of tiny lightning flashes. Both the frequency and power of these lightning storms can vary, depending on their locations in our brains, what we're doing at the time, and the particular challenges embedded in our individual hardware. Scientists depict the activity with images known as brain waves, the speed of which is measured in cycles per second, or hertz.

The theory behind neurofeedback is that our mental states correlate with whatever frequency is dominant, i.e., registering the highest voltage in our brains. Faster isn't necessarily better—slower waves, such as the so-called theta speeds of 4–8 Hz, can indicate an imagination at work. Still, most of us get through the day on faster beta waves, ranging from 12 Hz to as high as 35 Hz and correlating with mental states ranging from alert and relaxed to nervous and cranky. The next highest frequencies, gamma waves, are associated with bursts of concentration, problem-solving, and deep meditation.

We all need a variety of frequencies, just like we need all the keys of a piano. Still, many people stumble through life with a mismatch of resources to task. Kerson's video games are theoretically going to help tune up our brains by encouraging the right sorts of brain waves and inhibiting the less desirable ones. She also says she plans to "amplify" and "synchronize" parts of our brains, eliminating "static" and improving efficiency. It all sounds promising, and, after all, how risky could a non-invasive procedure be? Besides, I've checked around, and Kerson has some of the most impressive qualifications of anyone in northern California. Not only was she elected head of the membership society, she was trained by the field's illustrious founding father of the clinical field: M. Barry Sterman, professor emeritus of neurobiology and biobehavioral psychiatry at the University of California at Los Angeles Medical School.

She assures us that Buzz's map shows he has "textbook ADD" and that his brain should be "a fairly easy fix."

"He would really benefit from this," she says. "He should be more calm in his brain, more optimized, better able to attend to cognitive tasks."

"Less impulsive?" I ask.

"Yes, absolutely."

"Less oppositional?"

"There's a good chance."

"He'll stop hitting his brother?"

"Probably."

"Can you get him to start doing the dishes?"

"Let's not get carried away!"

I'm encouraged, however. I need to be, especially considering this: after a full year in which Buzz has been taking his meds, Jack and I want to give him a drug-free summer. What that means is that Kerson and her electrodes may be all that's standing between us and the return of Mr. Hyde.

SO, WHAT AM I, *nuts?*

After all the good the meds have done for Buzz and our family, why stop now? Am I just second-guessing away because I *can,* since with Buzz's improved behavior, the balance has finally shifted away from "better short than dead"?

I'm still a firm believer in the biological model of clinical distraction. The problem is I'm still not resigned, nor is Jack, to the meds-for-life approach. Prescription drugs in general may be much safer than their fiercest critics allege, but they're still by no means risk-free. In her book *Our Daily Meds,* Melody Petersen reports that they account for 270 U.S. deaths a day—more than twice as many as in car accidents. Part of the problem is that we Americans, bombarded as we are by all those cheery TV ads, are steadily increasing our use of all kinds of medications, and often combining them in risky ways.

I'm worried in particular about all the potential side effects from stimulants. I want to give Buzz a chance to grow taller, if he can, and I'm haunted by reports of how these meds can raise heart rates and blood pressure, even by small amounts. Chronic high blood pressure can sap the strength of organs like the heart and kidneys. Won't these small increases add up over time? Especially given the higher doses of stimulants kids are ingesting, due to all those longer-acting medications? Pelham, the research psychologist, has calculated that children who take these meds over the course of several years will ingest as much as thirty times the amount of methylphenidate prescribed barely a decade ago.

Maybe some risks are worth taking in return for guaranteed benefits. But just this past year, published reports have raised serious questions about whether the stimulants pay off after the first few years. In a three-year follow-up to that pivotal 1999 finding that methylphenidate was the single most effective treatment for ADD, the same federally sponsored researchers checked back and found that the initial advantage they'd detected was no longer apparent. The kids who'd been taking medication were just as vulnerable to the projected "bad outcomes" of delinquency, dropouts, and social failures.

Researchers conceded they weren't sure about the reasons for these discouraging results, even as they noted that many of the children who were being treated with medication alone during the study simply stopped taking their drugs after it ended. The implication was that in an ideal world, the kids would take their medicine faithfully, keeping their symptoms under control. Yet this remains an extremely idealistic view. On average, experts report, American kids stay on ADD meds no more than eighteen months, federal study or no federal study, after which inertia often kicks in. And this unfortunate rule applies not only to clinically distracted kids but to people with many other chronic conditions. Even *cancer patients,* whose lives may depend on faithfully taking their meds, often tire of the side effects or the routine, and quit.

I, too, became a stimulant slacker, following my own Ritalin honeymoon. After my first few months on methylphenidate, I no longer enjoyed that revved-up feeling, worried every time I felt what seemed to be a chest pain, got tired of and embarrassed about having to check in with a psychiatrist to keep getting prescriptions, and by the time Buzz started his drug "holiday," had reduced my use to just every once in a while.

If *I* can't stay the course, I figure, how can I expect Buzz to do so, as a teen or, especially, once he reaches adulthood? We both clearly need an alternative, assuming one exists.

I've been briefing Jack on all this during the rare moments we can talk out of earshot of the kids. But by tacit agreement, we haven't shared the details with Buzz, just as we didn't involve him in our original decision to start the meds. I wish Buzz could make his own decisions about the trade-offs he's willing to assume, yet of course it wouldn't be fair to flood an adolescent with such complex, contradictory, and changing information. And while it may not be quite fair to do that to an adult, either, the buck stops with us. Which is why, on the first day of summer vacation, Buzz is surprised to see there's no little yellow pill on his breakfast plate.

"Where's the pill?" he asks.

"We thought we'd take a break for the summer," I say, in a deliberately flat tone. "What do you think?"

"Sure!"

So we're good. For now.

ON A SIZZLING June afternoon, Buzz and I are back in separate rooms at Cynthia Kerson's office, for our third joint treatment session. Electrodes are stuck to our heads and clipped on our ears with a viscous goop that's hard to wash out and ends up staying in our hair for days. Kerson walks back and forth between us, checking the monitors.

By now we know the drill. Kerson places the electrodes according to what she says our brain maps tell her about where we need tuning up. We breathe in and try to relax so that our brains can respond to the feedback. Buzz is putting together a puzzle of a giant panda on his computer monitor. I've got the more "adult" job of focusing on a horizontal blue bar, which shrinks when I get it right. The better we do, the more the computer makes a pleasant *boop-boop-boop* sound, egging us on. As Kerson has explained it, our brains start out with fairly random behavior but learn to respond to that rewarding sound that starts in the moment we do it right—just like me "catching Buzz being good."

The theory behind this, and all biofeedback, is called operant conditioning, which means that as you get rewarded for a certain behavior, you behave that way more often. And it certainly fits right in with all I've been learning about Buzz and appreciation. Feed a dog just once from the table, and you can count on that dog begging at every future meal. Give your child effusive praise, or candy or cash, at the moment you see him pick up a sock, and you may just have a clean floor for days to come.

The difficulty is that the reverse is also true: Negative feedback can encourage nasty behavior. As I've been focusing on giving Buzz more positive feedback over the past few months, I've noticed Jack getting into more battles. That's partly because he's been spending more time with the kids, which offers more opportunities for squabbles. But he's also not quite getting this reinforcement magic, not so far at least. So, frequently, when Buzz or Max misbehave, Jack responds in kind.

"You . . . *knuckleheads!*" he said, at the end of his rope the other evening, after they'd sniped at each other all through dinner.

The feedback was instantaneous.

"*That's* not nice!" Max complained—never mind that he had just called Buzz a "retard."

"Yeah, some role model!" Buzz chimed in.

They badgered Jack, delightedly, for days about the "knuckleheads" comment, which they took as a license to call him names in return—terrible names, like "fatso" and "old codger." The tension built up until an evening on which I left Jack in charge while I snuck out for dinner with my friend Katy, during which, as was reported to me later, Max changed the channel on Jack's baseball game three times in a row, the last time spitefully fiddling with the remote so that Jack had to spend a couple of extra seconds getting back to where he'd been, and missed an important at-bat.

You can fiddle with Jack's bank account, his wardrobe, even his food. But you don't fiddle with the remote. Jack was so beside himself that he put his face close to Max's and shouted . . . "CHA-CHA-CHEEH!" No one, least of all Jack, knows what "cha-cha-cheeh" means, but it's now our family code word for Jack losing it.

"Mom is more patient than Dad," Buzz began saying around this time.

I'd certainly like to believe that all I've worked so hard to learn is starting to pay off. Even so, back in my darkened room at Kerson's office, it's starting to bug me that Buzz is doing so much better at his task than I am. Try as I may, I can't shut out the tauntingly steady *boop-boop boop* sound from across the hall, so much faster than my own.

Alone in the darkened room, I scrunch up my face, imagining the two hemispheres of my brain moving closer together, as if to physically force that stupid horizontal bar to shrink. This doesn't help, and it helps even less when Kerson comes in and looks over my shoulder at the monitor, shaking her head.

Kerson makes me nervous even when I'm doing well. She's constantly catching me doing something I shouldn't, like absentmindedly touching the tight gold electrode clip on my ear. "Stop that!" she'll say. And while I know I can be oversensitive about this sort of thing, it's annoying, the way she'll tut-tut over how few points I've earned, and *then* imply *I'm* too focused on the points.

"For people like you, this is the hardest part," she says. "I don't want you to have any judgment."

No judgment? NO JUDGMENT?!

I try to remember how it felt when I momentarily got it right and the bar shrunk. But that doesn't work either, and I recall that Kerson has told me I'm not supposed to try. *It doesn't make sense! How do you try to not try?*

During the rare moments when I seem to get the hang of it, neurofeedback is at once easier and harder than meditation. Easier, because the machine keeps reminding me to stay on track. Harder, because I can't get away with letting my mind wander for the entire half hour. The damnable machine is keeping score.

Kerson leaves the room, after which Buzz comes in, smiling victoriously. He grabs my cell phone to call the dim sum place. The deal is he gets pork buns after every session, plus $1 for every one hundred points he racks up on his games. Early on, this seemed reasonable. I didn't expect him to get so good so fast. And of course he's refusing to renegotiate.

What's more, now he's pushing it on the dim sum. As I hear him asking for *two* orders of pork buns, plus hot 'n' sour soup, and shu mai noodles, my already pathetically slow rate of *boop-boop-boop*ing comes to a halt.

"Buzz, that's too much food!"

He acts as if he doesn't hear, and I'm torn between wanting to leap from my chair and grab the phone, and trying to rack up just a few more points in my last twenty seconds. This session is going to be my worst.

Kerson comes in again, checks out the screen, and frowns at me.

"Buzz has done better each time, but you've sort of stayed the same," she begins. "I'm wondering if we need another strategy. . . ."

Buzz interrupts: "Mom, let's go! The Chinese dude said it'll be ready in fifteen minutes."

I keep my eyes on the screen. *C'mon, you freaking horizontal bar! Ten seconds to go!*

"You have to maybe give some thought to why you're like this," Kerson is saying, ignoring Buzz. "You seem much more attached to the outcome than I'd even thought. You're getting in the way of yourself."

I look up, nod vigorously, and smile—the kind of smile where you just use your mouth and not your eyes.

Back in the car, I ask Buzz about his technique.

"I just thought about how with all the dollars I'm going to get, I could buy a gecko!" he says.

"Oh, so *you* can be attached to the outcome!" I say.

I'm actually starting to miss the straightforward simplicity of the Ritalin Wars.

I TRULY LIKE and admire Cynthia Kerson, but we're not an easy match. The two of us are always in a rush—I need to drive Buzz to his Hebrew tutor right after the session, while she has other patients waiting. Plus I'm frustrated by not doing better at this, and not understanding it nearly well enough. I realize she's ultra-busy, dividing her time between raising two daughters, running her practice, travel-ing around as director of that membership group, and getting her PhD in "Applied Psychophysiology" through a distance-learning pro-gram based at the University of Natural Medicine in Santa Fe. She probably thinks I'm a pest, asking the same questions two or three times in a session, instead of trying to figure it out by myself.

So the atmosphere is already charged when we have yet another awkward conversation.

After looking at my brain map, Kerson tells me that she doesn't believe I have attention deficit disorder, after all. I just don't match the profile, she says. "How do you feel when I tell you that?" she asks. I've told her about my book project, my dream of a healing journey with Buzz.

"Um, I dunno," I say, mentally scrambling. *Does this mean I need to rethink the book? Or is it simply one more controversial opinion about an extraordinarily controversial disorder?* I fill out the scorecard: *Dr. Y., my shrink, thinks I have it. My husband Jack is sure I have it. My mother, father, and psychiatrist sister Jean lean more toward Kerson's view, but Dr. Daniel Amen's brain scan supposedly proves I have it. And now here's this QEEG. . . .*

I remind myself that psychiatrists diagnose ADD according to a checklist of symptoms, all of which Buzz and I unquestionably share. And also that girls' ADD supposedly usually manifests itself as some-thing else, like depression or anxiety.

"It's that kind of disorder, isn't it?" I finally murmur. "It's pretty confusing. So what do you think I do have?"

"The key to your issues is not inattention but fear."

"Mmhmm."

Well here, I'll agree. I've been anxious ever since I can remember, and am certainly extra anxious about Buzz. *And global warming.*

Kerson goes on to say I've got an "overaroused" brain, with a lot of high beta, which she would like to try to inhibit.

I consider her analysis for a day or two and then figure, what the heck. Whatever she wants to call my glitch, I wouldn't mind getting some help in calming down. And as more weeks go by, I keep faith in her approach, maybe because I really am getting a bit less reactive, but mostly because—is it my imagination?—after twenty sessions, Buzz may be getting easier to live with. He's still melting down a lot, but maybe less often; still hitting Max, but possibly less hard. And, no doubt about this: he's getting up easier in the mornings.

BUT THIS IS SO WRONG!

It's mid-July, on a sweltering late afternoon, and I've brought Buzz into my last refuge, my backyard shed, and turned it into hell.

As I've grown increasingly nervous over the way we're hemorrhaging money, what with the neurofeedback on top of the rapidly escalating costs of my remodeling project, I've rented equipment from Kerson, in an effort to cut down our bills by doing some of our sessions at home. She has given me a ninety-minute crash course, at her own kitchen table, on how to use her BrainMaster software, but I think I've missed some essentials, because lots of things are going wrong, all at once. There's conductive goop all over my hands, the EEG gizmo, the phone, and, somehow, Buzz's nose. I'm on my fourth attempt to attach an electrode to his left mastoid bone, but it keeps falling off, and I can no longer make sense of my notes from Kerson, scrawled on the brain map I've taped to my wall. From what I can decipher, the electrode with the blue wire is supposed to go on the area marked on the map as T6, midway down on the right side of the back of Buzz's head, while the red wire electrode goes on T5, on the other side, but what about the black and green wires? Kerson has instructed me to use a different setup for myself, which requires me to change the way these two wires are plugged into the gizmo. I've written "switch black and green" on Buzz's map, but am no longer sure what that means. Switch them for me? Have I already switched them?

The air outside is smoky. There are close to eight hundred wildfires raging around Sonoma County, within an hour's drive of our house. There are always wildfires in summer, but never like this, my friends and I say to one another, as we cough. *Armageddon . . . just a matter of time . . .*

"This is taking too long!" Buzz complains, and sneezes. He turns his face to wipe his nose on my bare arm as I lean over him, behind his chair.

"Stop that! Hold on, goddammit!" I say, pinching the clip on his ear, just a little too hard.

"Ouch! Hey!"

I finally get all the electrodes stuck in place, but now something else has gone awry. The waves on the monitor are jagged, saw-toothed, nothing resembling the smooth curves that indicate a clear signal. The *boop-boop-boop*ing has begun, but it's much too fast to be working correctly. Buzz is laughing now, anticipating extra points—and dollars—while typing on the laptop, changing the names of the icons on the screen. It now says "POOPY" where it used to say "BrainMaster," and he's moving on to write "HUGE DUMP" on the file I titled "Neurofeedback Log."

I'm hyperventilating.

I mean, right now. Even as I try to recapture this scene on paper, I'm hyperventilating.

While Kerson has assured me that many neurofeedback clients have great results with sessions at home, I'll later learn that it's not a universally accepted practice. Too many things can go wrong, as we've been finding out. Hair gets stuck under the electrodes. Electrodes break. Mysterious but urgent warnings flash on the screen relating to things like "WRONG COM PORTs." Trolling the Web, I discover an article in the *Journal of Neurotherapy*, warning of dire scenarios when neurofeedback goes wrong: tics, depression, "mental fogginess," seizures, panic attacks, incontinence . . .

Now Max comes out to the shed and presses his face against the glass door. "Can I try? Let me try!" he pleads. To him, this must look like a game, one more fun thing Buzz gets to do because of his lucky disorder. I turn, mustering a smile. "Hold on, sweetie, I'll be with you in just a sec!" *I'll have to make this up to him. But I'm already taking him to the violin camp next week. Isn't that enough? Shouldn't that be enough?* . . . Turning back to the computer, I see what appears to be a big gob of snot on the keyboard.

That's my limit: A helpless roar arises from somewhere deep inside of me: "Ohhhh, *CRAP!*"

"Mommy, you scared me!" shouts Max, from behind the door.

FOUR DAYS LATER, I'm sprawled on the sand in a cove along the Point Reyes seashore, picking at the last bits of mozzarella stuck to an empty pizza box.

The boys, at least for a few golden moments, have been playing peacefully together in my friend Katy's kayak. *Did I just hear Max say "jellyfish"?* Katy has not only invited us out here for the afternoon, but is also listening compassionately as I recount our nightmare in the shed. I've sought her advice after reading a long magazine story she wrote on neurofeedback, which to my delight included an honest assessment of her own lifelong problem with distraction. She'd careened between "ribbons and demerits," she wrote, acing her SATs and winning admission to Sarah Lawrence College, yet leaving behind a wake of minor car accidents, exasperated tax accountants, and friends hurt by things she'd blurted out. She'd tried "talk therapy," Ritalin, and seven months in a Buddhist monastery, but assured me nothing helped more than neurofeedback, which she maintained had made her less self-doubting and obsessive, and better able to sleep soundly, meet deadlines, and pack for trips.

The breakthroughs weren't immediate, nor did they come easy. Some practitioners gave her free treatments, while, to save money, she also, like me, tried some sessions at home. She wasted a lot of time, and says some sessions left her worse off than before. After one, she sat dazed in her hammock for three days, while another left her chewing furiously on a huge wad of gum. Why, she asked herself, had she let people she hardly knew put a Mixmaster into her brain?

I can answer that one. Neurofeedback's heady promise of lasting self-transformation, right down to your brain cells, in thirty to forty sessions, is seductive enough to have fueled a rapidly growing industry. I'm certainly still hopeful, although I'm ready to take a break from Kerson. Rightly or wrongly, I've lost some confidence after the debacle in the shed, while Buzz has been getting bored with her software and fighting about going to any more appointments.

Katy suggests we try out her favorite two local therapists, who share a practice: Jan Davis, a psychologist and former Montessori teacher, and Penel Thronson, a former psychiatric nurse. Under their electrodes, she says, "I suddenly saw how other people must feel all their lives . . . as if I'd had a nurturing childhood." Another plus: their office is just down the street from Buzz's favorite pizza parlor. That's enough for me. I call them the next day, and Buzz and I get an appointment within the week. We like them as soon as we meet them. They're both in their fifties, with short blond hair, and work out of the ground floor of their wood-shingled house full of books and Asian art. After interviewing me and reviewing our brain maps, Thronson offers a succinct explanation for what's been going wrong. "He's provocative," she says, "and you're reactive."

She and Davis assure me they can continue Buzz's treatment for distraction and oppositional behavior, while helping me slow down enough to have more of a choice about how I'll react—to Buzz and the rest of the world. "You'll get more space in your mind—a buffer," Thronson says. In an introductory session, they hook me up to one of their software programs for half an hour. Instead of a horizontal bar, it shows a forest scene that comes alive with greenery, butterflies, and birds when I manage to slow down but stay alert. The two women stay in the room with me during the session, making encouraging noises. It feels easier and better right away. I float through the rest of the afternoon and resolve to return for more sessions—as soon as I can find more time and money. For now, however, I need to focus on Buzz. It's mid-August, with barely a month to go before he becomes a bar mitzvah.

BUZZ FOLDS A PIZZA SLICE, closes his eyes, and savors his first bite, the cheesy juice dripping down his chin and probably permanently staining his new white polo shirt. I breathe in, from the diaphragm, and choose not to comment. We're sitting outside at that pizza parlor

down the street from Davis and Thronson's office, on an early evening in the first week of September, the sun slanting through pines
on a forested hill above the town. This place is so popular that people
are already lining up to wait. The service is slow, but it doesn't help,
does it? to be nervous about how late I'm going to be to pick up Max,
who's hanging out at a friend's house.

Buzz started eighth grade last week. He's had ten sessions with
Davis and Thronson so far, on top of the ones he had with Kerson,
and we plan to keep them up, twice a week after school, for at least
the next month or two. It's probably helpful that I now drop Buzz off
and get out of the way, using the time to take a walk or do errands,
since I'm putting off my own sessions for now. No more competing,
and I think Buzz also behaves better when I'm not around. He's doing
two sessions at a time now, spending up to fifty minutes at once,
which feels more efficient and may also be more effective.

Thronson reports that he's unusually cooperative. And there are
definitely more signs of progress at home: there are even fewer and
less intense meltdowns; he's fighting a bit less with Max, and he also
seems to be directing a lot, if not, alas, all, of the energy he once put
into bugging me to buy him things into healthier outlets. I've put a
basketball hoop in his room—one of the smartest things, by the way,
I've ever done—and he'll often shoot hoops there for an hour or
more. Sometimes he'll even go there in the middle of an argument,
as if giving himself a time-out. On top of this, he'll do these amazing
things every once in a while, like run up to me with crumbs all over
his face and a box of cookies I've unsuccessfully hidden, saying,
"Hide them again!"

I've checked in with his teachers and haven't heard of any serious
problems with attention. So far, so good. But one thing remaining un-
changed is his unwillingness to talk openly about any of this with me.

"Buzz, do you feel like you're having any improvements from the
neurofeedback?" I ask him.

He finishes chewing his pizza, slowly. "I guess so."

"No, really." I keep my voice steady. "You think it's making any
difference?"

"I guess so. . . ."

"What kind of difference is it making?"

A diabolical smile. "I guess so."

"Buzz, have you ever heard the phrase 'passive aggressive'?"

"I guess so."

There may never come a time when Buzz stops getting such pleasure from frustrating me, but as he gets slightly less intense about it, while I simultaneously work on being less frustrate-able, we're starting to enjoy each other's company more. We play Ping-Pong together—he has gotten so good that he'll do these showboat moves like spinning himself around while waiting for my return, and I'll *still* lose the point—and a deceptively simple board game called Othello, and I'm still reading to him at night. Buzz seems to like himself better, so he likes me better, too. "You're the greatest mom ever!" he writes on a card that I immediately tape to my office wall.

I'm proud of him for hanging in there with this effort to improve himself, no matter how much he still tries to make me pay for his points at every session. And along the way, I realize my initial goal for this process has changed dramatically. At first I'd hoped the neurofeedback would "cure" Buzz's attention problems, the same hope I'd had for the pill. But as he gets easier to live with, I'm starting to realize that this new agreeableness is really what I've most wanted. Besides, if Buzz continues to be less oppositional, maybe he'll start taking responsibility for coping with his own problems, finding his own ways to compensate for and get the best from a flickering mind.

How much is the neurofeedback really helping? There's no real way to know. Maybe he's just finally starting to mature, his brain catching up with his chronological age. Still, I feel sure there's more to it than that, even if it's merely the way we've adapted our lives to invest in this new treatment. Cliff Saron, my neuroscientist friend, has a term for this phenomenon, which he applies to his research on the impact of meditation retreats. He calls it the *tuchus* effect, representing the sheer fact of putting your *tuchus* on a mat, day after day, to the exclusion of other things you'd been doing. By choosing to go on a meditation retreat, you also choose to leave your busy life, travel somewhere, simplify your routine, eat regular meals, and cooperate with a group of other, like-minded people. It's the same with Buzz and me and neurofeedback. We have more than the *boop-boop-boop*ing. We also have all the time we're spending driving to and fro, eating pizza, and talking about our expectations, as we share this vision of more calm and focused lives.

Gene Arnold, who's leading that new federally sponsored research project on neurofeedback for attention deficit disorder, shares my suspicion that there's much more to the experience than what happens in the practitioner's office. "Almost any problem will improve if you pay attention to it," he says. "These kids are coming in two to three times a week with their parents, probably stopping at McDonald's, getting all that quality time, with the parents expecting them to do better—it's bound to make a difference."

Added to this, as I've already mentioned, Arnold has faith the actual brain-wave training can also make a difference. And yes, so do I. Not least because just the other day, when I was waiting in line at the post office, flustered and running behind schedule, as usual, I suddenly remembered the image of that flowering forest from Davis and Thronson's software.

In my mind, I heard the *boop-boop-boop*. And I felt better, really better, right away.

CHAPTER 9

MEDITATION

"No One Ever Died of Restlessness"

*For one who has trained the mind,
the mind is the best of friends.
For one who has failed to train the mind,
the mind is the greatest enemy.*

BHAGAVAD GITA

THE CLOCK ON MY DASHBOARD READS 5:29 P.M. AS I VEER OFF onto the country road heading into the hills above the town of Woodacre, home of the Spirit Rock Meditation Center. Only one minute left before the deadline to appear for my five-day retreat.

It's the Wednesday before Labor Day, and another insanely hot afternoon, the temperature exceeding one hundred degrees. *Instead of indulging in this navel-gazing marathon, I should be planning a move to some place with a healthier climate, and preferably also without an impending earthquake. . . .*

The Spirit Rock retreat center sits in a valley amid 410 acres of stunningly beautiful undeveloped land—shady oak woodlands and golden, Andrew Wyeth–y rolling hills—purchased from the Nature Conservancy in 1987. *California's oak woodlands are one of the planet's most endangered ecosystems, threatened by development, climate change, and competition from invasive species.* The center has hosted such world-famous Buddhist teachers as Jack Kornfield, one of its founders; Thich Nhat Hanh; and Ram Dass. Hundreds of people attend classes and retreats here every week.

As I turn into the parking lot, I pass a large yellow sign urging me to "YIELD to the Present."

As *if.*

My mind is churning, as usual, over worries large and small, including how the heck I'm going to figure out the guest count for Buzz's bar mitzvah, given that I forgot to include RSVP cards when I sent the invitations. And how I'm going to pay the caterer, in light of our bank's unexpected reluctance to increase our equity loan. . . .

5:34 P.M. *Damn! Late again!* And only because I stopped to buy a cup of coffee on the way, a kind of formal, temporary adieu to artificial stimulants. I feel like Paris Hilton, checking into detox. *Whose crazy idea was this, anyway? Oh, right: Cliff Saron's.*

"You should go on a silent, five-day retreat," my neuroscientist friend said, like a doctor prescribing a drug, shortly after I failed that awful sustained-attention test in Colorado. In subsequent weeks, he pressed the point, e-mailing me abstracts of scientific studies illuminating various ways in which meditation, or "mindfulness," may improve focus and curb impulsivity, particularly for hard cases like me.

Researchers suggest that entire families can benefit if even one person regularly meditates, since that person may then help defuse other members' hotheadedness. This more than anything persuaded me that dedicating five days to doing not much of anything while Jack takes off work to handle the grocery shopping, cooking, laundry, errands, and child care, will be my special gift to *him. Yeah, that's the ticket!*

The catch, of course, is that those who stand to benefit the most from meditation usually have the hardest time actually doing it. "It sounds promising, and really makes sense," the ADD expert Dr. Russell Barkley told me, when I collared him after his talk in Davis. "But these are people who have trouble following through on everything. . . ."

I'm not all *that* bad. I've been married for twenty years and held on to a job for almost the same amount of time. Yet it's certainly also true that I've never kept up with piano practice, leave parties when they're just getting started, and too often even tune out in the middle of a conversation. Being a reporter has been my best excuse. *I'm just an observer. I need to go call my editor.* And when it comes to meditation, despite all my good intentions, I've at best maintained a foxhole practice. I'll count breaths late at night to ward off a panic attack. But take time away from work? On a regular basis? Not so far. And stop everything—even talking—to sit around for five days? *What was I thinking?*

Still, I wish Dr. Russell Barkley could see me now, determinedly hauling my wheeled suitcase up the hill to the redwood-paneled dorms. Over the past couple of weeks, I've put off work deadlines, hired a sitter from an expensive agency, convinced three mothers to host sleepovers, and gotten Jack's okay after delivering a speech that included the phrase "cancer survivor."

Buzz has watched my preparations bemusedly. Last night, in the kind of friendly gesture he's making more often these days, he hid a walkie-talkie handset under the pillow on my bed, making it *SQUAWK* just as I was settling back with the newspaper.

"So what will you actually do there? Over!" he asked, from his room.

"You know, meditate. . . . Over!"

"You really can't talk to anyone? Over!"

"Well, that's the rule. It's a silent retreat. Over!"

"No talking? No e-mail? No TV? That doesn't sound like much of a life, Mom! Over!"

"I know. I'm pretty scared I'll get bored. Over!"

"If you get bored, will you come home early? Over!"

I assured Buzz I wouldn't, but I'm nonetheless marveling over how I've now made it all the way to the registration desk without racing back to my car. Greeting the arrivals is a woman wearing a headband with faux ocelot ears. "*You* look athletic," she tells me with a smile.

My karma for looking athletic is a "work meditation" assignment to the lunchtime, dining-hall chair-stacking and mopping crew. *What a scam!* my reporter-mind clicks on to announce. *There are, let's see, eighty-seven privileged white folk here, paying $600 a head,* *while the retreat managers not only don't have to pay for meat, alcohol, or desserts, but are saving on labor!*

But then I notice the large sign on the registration table. "The BUDDHA," it reads, "teaches to receive whatever room and food is offered with gratitude and a bow."

I smile back at the woman with the ocelot ears.

STILL WEDNESDAY. 7:30 P.M. I sit cross-legged, then change position to kneel on my pillow, then cross my numb legs again, sneaking a look at my watch. It's our very first forty-five minutes of sitting meditation, and, just as I'd feared, I'm already blowing it. Slowing down abruptly from full speed ahead isn't coming naturally; about five minutes after I closed my eyes to try to focus on my breath, I fell asleep, jerking awake with a start. And now my thoughts are snagging on such minor details as the license plate resting on the backseat of my car. I got new license plates last week and, for reasons I'm not sure I can explain, only had time to screw in the one on the front of the car. Then I got distracted, after which I couldn't find the screwdriver. . . . *Why is this so hard, anyway? It's just sitting.* But it brings me back to when I was a restless kid, and my mother, a bit anxious herself, would say, "Do something constructive!" This just doesn't feel constructive enough.

The woman to my right—lean and disciplined, at least twenty years younger than me, and wearing a tight orange T-shirt that says something about Nepal—appears to be stifling a smile. *Dear God, or Buddha, please let me not have snored.* I just need to hang on for fifteen more minutes until the "dharma talk," after which I can slink off to bed. . . .

Surveys suggest that more than 10 million Americans are meditating these days. Public school teachers are coaching students to count their breaths; Kaiser Permanente is offering classes in "mindfulness-based stress reduction"; moms picking up their grade school kids are sporting Sanskrit tattoos; and engineers at Google, that global hub of distraction, are getting on-the-job contemplative training. The fourteenth Dalai Lama of Tibet has had two books, simultaneously, on the *New York Times* best-seller list, and even Lisa Simpson, the cartoon character, has converted to Buddhism.

Boosting the trend is the modern notion that meditation offers healthy mental exercise, a means of not only fending off stress but also working out those focus muscles that start failing in midlife. Many modern gurus encourage this brain-fitness paradigm, suggesting, in the words of the monk and author Matthieu Ricard, that a meditative regimen might be seen as more like going to a gym than "blissing out under a bongo tree."

Spirit Rock's approach is measurably more devout than this model, yet far from ascetic. The rooms, while spare, are comfortable, with two roommates at the most; the food, if bland, is light on the tempeh; and the rules are flexible. Each sitting session, in the high-ceilinged meditation hall, with its gleaming wooden floors and gold statues of the Buddha, lasts less than an hour, and no one thwacks you with a stick if you change position. It's up to us whether to count our breaths, silently recite a mantra, or simply try to stay aware. During the day, we alternate between periods of sitting and walking meditation, in which we place one foot in front of the other as slowly and deliberately as possible. There's also a daily yoga class, for even more variety.

Between the chimes of the gong that mark the start and end of our five days of Noble Silence, we're not supposed to talk. But cheats are allowed during the work meditations and if we need to communicate with staff members.

I needed to communicate with a staff member soon after I arrived, since I'd forgotten to pack a towel and was looking to rent one. Alone in the administrative office with the employee, whom I'll call Shelly, I took the opportunity to whisper—it felt less like cheating that way—a question about how Spirit Rock compares with most of the other Buddhist retreats popping up around the country. I'd already heard that in traditional Zen centers, you're expected to show up at four-thirty in the morning, and you eat your meals while sitting on your meditation pillow.

Shelly had spent the last two hours dealing with several other special requests for extra towels, blankets, pillows, and socks, which may explain why she answered as she did. She confided that she worried about all the laxity and comfort, adding, "You can't simultaneously seek enlightenment and the perfect croissant."

I nodded at this, but frankly didn't share her concern. Enlightenment would be great, but my dearest hope was to get enough out of this week to last *one day* back home without getting into a fight. Or losing my sunglasses. Or keys. Or cell phone. . . .

Our teachers raise my expectations. "By the time you leave here, your hearts will be more tender, and your view will be more clear," promises Howard Cohn, during the night's dharma talk. Cohn is movie-star good-looking—tall, curly haired, and gray-eyed—which seems as vaguely inappropriate as the semiprivate rooms. "You're cooling your reactivity, with every minute of mindfulness making you less contentious," he tells us. "I can't think of any greater gift you can give yourself and the people around you."

I write this last part down eagerly, looking forward to reading it to Jack when I get back.

"KU-MII-ORII, KIVA-AH ORAYYICHHH!"

That's Hebrew, a line Buzz has supposedly been memorizing for his upcoming bar mitzvah by listening to our synagogue's Cantor David sing it on a CD we play on the car stereo every time I drive him anywhere. Now it's stuck in my head.

"Arise! Shine! For your light has dawned! The Presence of the Lord has shone upon you!"

I hear Cantor David bellowing in my mind soon after I wake to my roommate's alarm clock at 5:15 A.M. I hear him again as I sprinkle chili flakes on my tofu at lunch, desperate for any semblance of excitement, and as I hike in the woodlands in the afternoon. But I hear him most reliably each time I settle down to try to meditate.

It's Thursday, Day 1, another sweltering late afternoon, and I'm kneeling on my pillow, trying to keep my back straight, clear my mind of all that Hebrew, and not dwell on what I might be catching from the woman behind me, who has what doctors describe as a "productive" cough.

People breathe heavily to my right and left. *This must be what it's like to be a sheep or cow: huddled close, bored, breathing, waiting for the next meal.*

My tailbone is on fire. And this business of staying motionless but awake isn't getting any easier, especially in the afternoon heat. I've fallen asleep in *three* of today's sitting sessions so far, each time returning to consciousness after only a minute or two, with an embarrassing jerk of my head. Back home, I'd fantasized about five whole days of simplicity, and being responsible only for myself. Now that I'm here, I can't wait to leave. *Twenty-four hours is enough, isn't it? Twenty-four hours is so much more than I've ever done before!*

At last the gong sounds, and I stagger to my feet, my legs angrily prickling back to life. With fifteen minutes before dinner, I head for the bench outside the dining hall to write a couple of pages in my notebook. I've skipped three of the sitting sessions—to sleep in, hike, and take a long shower—my guilt only somewhat relieved by noting how many other retreatants I've seen are doing the same thing.

At dinner, however, when we're all here in the same room, everyone seems to be fully participating in what's known as "mindful eating"—the practice of silently keeping our attention fixed on the food.

"Mindful eating is a wonderful context for the arising of insights," say the Spirit Rock retreat rules, which I read on the Internet last week. "The simple, mindful eating of an apple connects us to the orchard far away from our dining table, to the sun and rain and earth that nurture the tree, to the grower, the picker, the trucker, the grocer, to the truth of the interconnectedness of all existence."

Alas, my mind is full, but not with images of interconnectedness. It's not just the petty mental soundtrack—*Where'd she get those beans? I didn't see beans! Are some people getting special food? How can I get beans?* I also can't seem to resist exchanging subversive glances with a fellow retreat virgin named Chris, a professional opera singer with long dark hair and bright hazel eyes. I met her in the first hour after registration, when we were still allowed to talk, and now we'll catch sight of each other, glumly chewing our lentils, and trade flashes of irony, and then quickly look back at our plates, as if we're back in fourth grade.

Chris and I were supposed to be roommates. Before that first gong chimed, we were sitting on our hard twin beds, cheerfully discussing why we'd come. I told her about my son and my book, and she told me about her hope to clear her mind so as to face what she summarized as a classic midlife crisis. She won my heart by confiding that she, too, worried she wouldn't last all five days, saying: "I almost bolted just now when the parking lot guy asked if I'd mind being 'blocked in'!"

It was just a minute later, however, that Shelly, the staff person, poked her head in to ask if one of us might switch places with a woman who was allergic to the carpet in her assigned room. And I volunteered, which was probably wise, since Chris and I might otherwise have stayed up all night talking.

My new roommate was more reserved: slender and thirtyish, she wore a black knit dress that fit her perfectly. By the time I arrived, her clothes and towels were folded neatly on the shelf. We only had time for a perfunctory greeting, although I managed to tell her I was there for reasons related to attention deficit disorder.

"My *ex-boyfriend* had ADD," she retorted, with a look that implied this had something to do with why *she* was there. From that point on, we both rigorously observed the Noble Silence.

DAY 2: FRIDAY, 11 A.M. Eight of us sit on straight-backed wooden chairs in a small, stuffy room, entered from a passage alongside the meditation hall. We're here for our first group check-in. None of us make eye contact. Instead, we stare at our hands, or the door. We might as well be in a doctor's waiting room, anticipating bad news.

Cohn warned us in his dharma talk that by today, the second day, "stuff may come up"—bad memories, unresolved issues. Perhaps that includes this ferocious impatience I'm feeling, like fire-alarm bells warning that this whole endeavor is a shameful, self-indulgent waste of time. *People are starving. The planet is burning. And I'm hanging out with a bunch of overindulged nutjobs trying to perfect their slow strides!*

My restlessness boiled over yesterday during my first lunchtime work meditation, as I watched three guys, who looked *quite athletic,* assigned to slice zucchini into little fillips, while I strained my back hauling the heavy black floor mats from the kitchen to be washed in the steamy heat outside. On my own team, there were two other guys who spent most of their time slow-walking around with languid smiles while I huffed and puffed past. One, in his late thirties I'm guessing, kept pausing to reapply his sunscreen; the other, much younger, stopped for several minutes while holding his mop upside down and staring at it as if in a trance. *He's contemplating the mop!* I thought. *Oh, man, Chris would love that! Contemplating the mop!*

As I wait for the check-in, however, I marvel at what a strange luxury this is, after all, to have attention to spare to be bothered by the work-meditation crew. Life at home is even more harried than usual these days. With school out for summer, three full months of camp unaffordable, and so little structure to their lives, the boys are teasing each other like never before. Buzz called Max "fat" at the breakfast table last week, after which Max called Buzz a "retard," after which Buzz spit on Max's waffle, after which Max ran to the bathroom, grabbed Buzz's toothbrush, and wiped it on his butt.

"No more calling anyone 'retard,' or 'gay,'" I declared, blithely abandoning decades of personal reverence for freedom of speech.

"Okay, I'll call him 'fat,'" Buzz promptly responded.

"No 'fat.'"

"Okay, 'nipples.'"

"No 'nipples.'"

"Okay, 'napples.'"

At least there's been the small consolation of more sincere camaraderie from Jack, who has been continuing to spend more time with the boys, as I've been trying harder to step back. The other night, we were watching a rerun of a Morley Safer interview with the actress Helen Mirren on *60 Minutes*. Safer, looking compassionate, asked Mirren if she ever regretted not having had children.

"No," she replied matter-of-factly. "Absolutely not. Absolutely not. I am so happy that I didn't have children. Well, you know, because I've had freedom."

My eyes met Jack's across the room, the expression on both of our faces saying: *Remember the week on that beach in the Philippines? The jazz clubs in Rio? Sleeping late . . . ?*

Max intercepted the look.

"Hey, no fair!" he shouted.

In the check-in room, at least three of us have our eyes locked on the clock on the wall—our leader is eight minutes late—by the time Wes Nisker walks in, without any air of hurry or apology. As he takes his seat, he looks slowly at each of our faces, mutely establishing that he has all the time he needs to be that deliberate, and that maybe we do, too. He greets us in a solemn baritone, then asks: "How many people here have an agitated mind?"

And every hand goes up.

Each of us is anxiously impatient to tell Nisker how we'd suffered through yesterday, the first full day of our retreat.

One woman, who has been in two recent car accidents, complained that she couldn't keep her mind off her pain. A young man says his mind was so agitated that when he turned his attention to his breath, his breath got agitated, too. Another says he's disappointed that he still hasn't felt any bliss. "Where's the bliss?" he demands, as if he'd ordered it with his burger.

Nisker seems to wince. "It was just the first day," he says, wriggling his large features back to composure. "You understand that, don't you? No one gets liftoff on the first day."

Nisker is a former Bay Area radio journalist-turned-professional-entertainer. The *New York Times* has described him as the world's first Buddhist stand-up comedian, who makes "suffering a knee-slapper." Like Howard Cohn, Jack Kornfield, Cliff Saron, and, most recently, me, Nisker also belongs to a cultural phenomenon commonly referred to as Bu-Jews: seekers of solace who've been raised in a culture of exceptional angst. He jests that our special mantra should be "om, shalom."

In his decades of coping with his own agitated mind, Nisker sampled a smorgasbord of consciousness-raising techniques, from Rolfing to tantric sex, to men's drumming sessions, to lying on his back with a colored disk on his forehead. Nothing, he says, beat Buddhist meditation in helping to cope with the restlessness so fundamental to human nature.

He jokes about the thoughts that must have troubled cavemen:

"I don't like the color of my spear."
"Who's going on the hunt tomorrow?"
"Who's watching the fire?"

These days, he says, while the scripts have changed—we worry more about mortgages and 401(k)s—we're still writing little stories to busy our minds, distracting us from thoughts of inevitable loss and death.

"And then we go on retreat and pull out the binkie [the pacifier]—of planning and doing, and it makes us *very* restless," Nisker says. "Nothing's happening. There'll be a disaster! But no one has ever died of restlessness."

As I listen to him, my hands rest on my journal, an eight-by-ten hardback composition notebook, as it lies in my lap. A couple of other people have notebooks here: it's a time when it's supposedly okay to write. But I've been transgressing at other times, when, according to the retreat rules, I should have been trying to stay in the moment. I have an excuse: I'm here not only to try to evolve, but to report this chapter, while handicapped by a poor memory. Still, I can imagine what Nisker might say, and I know he'd be right: *the notebook is my binkie.*

While we can't change who we are, we can hope to change how we react, Nisker is telling the check-in group, adding that the beloved Buddhist teacher Ram Dass used to observe that years of meditation "never changed his personality. He just learned to see it as a pet."

Buddhists aren't alone in recognizing this particular wisdom. "We are disturbed not by what happens to us, but by our thoughts about what happens," noted the freed Greek slave Epictetus, circa 100 CE. And it's such a powerfully liberating thought: that it might one day be possible, say, with a lot of contemplation, neurofeedback, and maybe even a lobotomy, for it not to matter so much to me that other people on my work-meditation crew aren't working as hard as I am, or even that my kids are so wild.

At the dharma talk, a few hours later, I'm watching my room-mate's back, motionless and perfectly straight, as she sits in the front row. I have no idea how she does that; it's hard for me even to imagine. Cohn mentions that he has received several notes complaining about all the people who've been arriving late to the meditation sessions, noisily opening the heavy wooden doors and settling onto their cushions. The authors asked him to scold the slackers. "People are getting annoyed," he acknowledges. "But on the other hand, you might also think: Wow, the doors are opening again—more people are coming!"

STILL DAY 2: FRIDAY, 4 P.M. I'm a woman on a mission, walking briskly down the hill, past the wooden gate, with its sign that says, "Retreatants Only Past This Point." In my hand is a screwdriver, which I've just borrowed from Shelly at the administrative office. She didn't ask me why I needed it, which was lucky, because even I'm aware of the wackiness of my behavior. At every one of the sitting sessions today, I've been unable to keep my mind off the license plate in my back seat. I've simply got to do something about it.

While the retreat rules make no specific mention of trips to the parking lot, I feel fairly sure our teachers wouldn't approve. It seems like just the kind of distraction we're supposed to be able to notice, but not pursue. Why can't I hold out? I might as well be reaching for a bong, or yelling at the kids. Truly, I feel wretched about this.

And yet, and yet—taking care of that license plate makes me feel almost as good as I knew it would. I kneel in the dust, taking time with each screw, making sure the connection is firm. I'm resolving something, achieving something I can feel with my hands. It occupies less than three minutes, but they are rich and fruitful minutes: *constructive* minutes. Sighing contentedly, I stand to wipe some oak leaves off the windshield, and then just sit quietly in the front seat of the car for a while.

For good measure, I take out the coffee cup I've left in the drink holder. As I look for a trash can, heading back up the hill, I notice a small wooden hut I hadn't seen on the way down. It's a shrine, filled with old photographs of Kornfield, the Spirit Rock cofounder, and some of his teachers, in the forests of Thailand. I look closely at one of the portraits, of a laughing bald man sitting in a lotus position. A placard identifies him as the venerable Ajahn Chah Subhato, 1918–92, and includes this quote:

> Try to be mindful and let things take their natural course. Then your mind will become still in any surroundings, like a clear forest pool. All kinds of wonderful, rare animals will come to drink at the pool, and you will clearly see the nature of all things. You will see many strange and wonderful things come and go, but you will be still. This is the happiness of the Buddha.

Stillness. What a concept. What a beautiful, foreign concept. Keeping the monk's words in mind, I leave the hut and walk slowly up the hill back to the dormitories.

I grew up in a casually observant Jewish family, where I'd ceased to believe in a Charlton Heston sort of God by the time I was eleven. Even so, I'll still sometimes pray as if a spirit with an actual personality and even a sense of fairness can hear: *Don't let him get hurt. Don't let it be malignant. Don't let the climate fall apart at least until my great-grandchildren get to lead healthy lives.* Buddhism offers the alternative view that we ourselves have the power to determine the nature of our lives, and to become more as we'd imagine God to be: unruffled by change or the force of emotion. And it's so compelling. . . .

I'm interrupted here, however, as I see Chris, in front of the dining hall, her hair combed back in a ponytail under a baseball cap with the visor bent down over her eyes, like a spy. The minute she spots me, she looks theatrically to her right and left, and then hands me a folded-up note she has been carrying. By the weirdest of coincidences, *she has also just visited her car,* and even compounded the transgression by turning on the radio and *listening to the two o'clock news.*

"*I had to tell someone!*" says her note. "*John McCain just picked this unknown woman governor from Alaska as his running mate. She has NO political experience. His goose is cooked!*"

I ruminate about the presidential campaign for the next two hours, my thoughts racing between hope and fear. This is my normal MO, of course, yet the retreat may be working its magic, after all, because with so few other distractions, I've at least begun to notice the way my mind behaves, and how uncomfortable it is, and how much company I have in this particular kind of suffering, and how ready I am, finally, to try something new.

DAY 3: SATURDAY, 1 P.M. I'm hiking again, during our free hour after lunch. It's finally cooling off, with fog sweeping over the hills. Surprisingly, I've had a much easier time on my pillow today. I've gone to every meditation session and haven't fallen asleep once. I'm not worrying about that license plate anymore and also seem to have more mental energy, which of course may not be surprising in view of how much space I've freed from keeping track of Hebrew tutoring and swim practice and whether we're running out of oranges.

I start out on a new trail, which leads uphill behind the meditation hall, through a grove of oaks. After just a few minutes of walking, I come upon a large gray boulder where people have left mementos—pictures, letters, jewelry—of dead friends, relatives, and pets. There's a picture of a beautiful girl who died at eighteen, a dog tag, and a Mother's Day card for a woman who didn't get the chance to read it. "If we really knew how fleeting life is, we'd live different lives," her daughter has written.

Our teachers have been talking a lot about just this idea: how we need to keep in mind how we'll all die at some point; that we have only a limited number of present moments to embrace. Focusing on our breath, hour after hour, is another reminder: proof of how much we rely on something so fragile and mercurial. But this new reminder at the boulder leads me right to my next distracting obsession:

I have to call Jack and the kids to make sure they're okay.

Communication with the outside world is one of the biggest no-nos of the retreat. But now I can't get the thought out of my mind. How can I do this? There's no cell-phone reception here, and I don't want to drive off the grounds. And I sure can't use the phone in the office.

Or can I?

The evening dharma talk makes it worse. Our third teacher, a kind-looking, gray-haired woman named Anna Douglas, is talking about summoning compassion, encouraging us to start out by imagining the face of someone we love. "Think to that person: May you be safe," she instructs us. "May you be well. May you be happy. . . ."

I sneak a glance at the twilit sky, streaked with orange, through the large window to my right, and imagine Jack's face, and am suddenly winded by how much I love him. And how petrified I am that he'll suddenly vanish. *A heart attack, a car crash, a mugger, an earthquake . . .* Another image comes to mind, of our family as if from far away: four people stuck together like atoms in a molecule on the verge of splitting apart. The meditation teacher Joseph Goldstein praises the goal of "liberation through not clinging." *Man, I am so far from that.* It's almost hard to breathe, I so badly need to call home.

I skip the evening walking meditation to stroll over to the office, where I'm encouraged to see Shelly, who always seems so approachable, and who may even still remember and appreciate the way I gave up my room that first day. *She'll* understand. . . . But then I remember her quip about the croissant. *Why* should *she help? It wouldn't do* her *any good. Why shouldn't she see me as spoiled, stubborn, shamefully attached? Maybe she even knows how many meditation sessions I've skipped. . . .*

"Look, I know I'm not supposed to use the phone," I begin. "So I'm wondering if you might do it for me. I just want to let my husband know how grateful I am that he is holding down the fort while I'm here."

This is actually only partly true. I mostly want to make sure he's still alive.

Shelly looks at me with what seems like a trace of censure. *Just as I thought.* "Why don't you take the time to think about this a little?" she asks.

I meet her eyes and silently shake my head. *Been there, done that.*

As if slipping her a bribe, I write down Jack's number at the *Chronicle*, where, as I explain, he's working late tonight, and hand her the paper.

"I know it's wrong; I just can't help it," I whisper, smiling weakly, as I edge toward the door.

I walk back to the meditation hall under a moonless, cloudless sky, bright with stars. *I've wasted my time with Shelly. I'm probably wasting my time with the retreat. She'll probably just throw the paper away. Maybe she'll report me. After all, it's like I'm trying to make her commit a crime for me. . . . She must think I'm such a loser. . . .*

At least this is my favorite part of the day, the Sanskrit chanting before bedtime, in the hall lit only by a few small candles. *Om mani padme hum.* "The jewel is in the lotus. Compassion is in the heart." The melody is hypnotic, calming; the darkness, private and intimate. I stay until the end and then return to my room, where my roommate is already sleeping.

The next morning, as I pass the bulletin board outside the meditation hall, I almost miss seeing the note pinned there, with my name. It's from Shelly.

"Kathy, you are such a dear!" she writes. "Thank you for giving me the opportunity to express your loving gratitude to your husband. All is well and he sends his love. He was touched by your thoughtfulness."

Now, *that's* weird. I stand there, stunned, holding the note, as people move past me into the hall. There's a warmth spreading through my chest. This is like some Buddhist jujitsu, where the weight of all my terrible self-doubt has served to thrust me into an epiphany. Which is that Shelly, in her extraordinarily compassionate interpretation of my craven impulse, has shown me the true meaning of that overused Sanskrit greeting—*Namaste*. I've used that word so many times with dripping irony, poking fun at the groovy subculture. *Namaste,* you lotus-eaters! But here I am, face-to-face with its literal meaning: "the divine light in me honors the light within you." Shelly was willing to interpret my behavior in the most generous, compassionate way, even if it meant breaking a rule.

Sunday, Day 4, breezes by. I'm free from obsessions, at least for now, and meditating away. My shoulders seem to settle a few inches lower each time I exhale. It's almost pleasant. And I realize something that seems significant: paying close attention is like playing red light/green light with both lights on at the same time. Saying yes to focusing on my breath means saying no to worrying about the presidential campaign, or the tingling in my legs, or to wondering why I can't keep my back as straight as my roommate's. Just as William James suggested, I'm choosing my world, thought by thought. Here on retreat, of course, the choice is relatively simple; no one's knocking on my door, or expecting me to cook dinner. But there's a reason they call this practice: I'm getting a chance to try on this new way of being, and it's feeling increasingly less strange.

Then comes the dawn of Monday, when I wake for the first time before my roommate's alarm. There's an hour before the first meditation session, so I head for the hills to catch the sunrise.

It's still dark when I begin, but as I near the top of the hill, dawn is spreading up through the gap where a line of undulating hills meets the forested ridges overlooking the coast. A hawk screams, and I try not to think about mountain lions, as I watch the fog peel back from the highway below. It will be a year next week from the time Buzz had his coffee meltdown in the car, starting me on this journey. I watch the traffic for a few moments, tranquilly wondering what kind of dramas might be taking place inside each of the vehicles rushing below.

Later, back in the meditation hall, Howard Cohn tries to prepare us for reentry, still cheerleading away. "You'll be amazed at how much energy you have and how sensitive you are—and that your personality hasn't changed," he says.

The gong sounds. We can talk again. Chris and I seek each other out and frantically try to catch each other up on all the conversations we've had with each other in our imaginations. We're talking a mile a minute, which makes me feel both happy and nervous, as I immediately start to miss that calm veil of silence. But we're both clearly so proud of ourselves and each other for lasting; we deeply understand how hard it was. We chat about the election, but it isn't nearly as satisfying as I'd thought it would be, back when chatting was taboo.

I exchange a few words with my roommate, but only a few. She looks as if she has been crying, and I scold myself for having assumed she didn't need to be here just as much as I did. Then I run into the guy with the sunscreen, from the dining hall crew, whom I'd told myself was clearly so dainty and shallow. We yak away as if we're old friends, as he reveals that he's a hardworking lawyer who got interested in retreats after his father and brother died in the same year. He's also generous, if belatedly, with his experience. When I complain about how I kept falling asleep, he shakes his head. "They really should have given us some basic instructions," he says. "Next time, if that happens, pull on your ear."

THREE BLACK BANANAS covered with flies lie in a bowl on the kitchen counter. The toilet in the boys' bathroom is leaking, and stinking. I've got 125 new e-mails to read.

I'll get to it. . . . There's time.

Whoa! Who planted *that* friendly new voice in my head? And what's it been smoking? And while we're at it, who painted the sky? Is it just an especially beautiful day, or have I somehow not been noticing?

I sit with Jack and the boys out on the back porch. Max is standing behind me, hugging me and playing with my hair, as if he's making up for lost time. Buzz sits a few feet away, but smiles at me with what seems like genuine interest as I tell them all about the bright stars, the mountain lions, Chris's note, Shelly's phone call, and how happy I am to be home.

Then Jack, who has been waiting patiently, tells me he almost lost his job three days ago, on Friday. In the half week I've been gone, the *Chronicle* managers, in yet another round of cost-cutting and layoffs, have offered buyouts to a couple dozen people in the news-room, including Jack, who dodged the bullet only after the union in-tervened.

He draws the story out, watching my eyes, and ends with the kicker: "I needed you, and you weren't here."

Now, Jack and I may be more blunt with each other than many other long-married couples. It's probably our adaptation to knowing we're going to get interrupted at any time by some new emergency with Buzz, and having to make the most of the few moments we have. I don't usually mind it, but right now I'm sharply aware of the effort it is taking to notice, but not do anything about, the chorus of anxious thoughts that his words have evoked. *How manipulative! How dare he even suggest . . . ! Oh—but have I let him down? How could I have been so selfish? Does he still love me?*

I breathe in the late-summer sunshine, the drone of bees, the tickle of Max's hands in my hair, and marvel over how these old, fa-miliar thoughts haven't led me once again straight to the nightmare scenarios of heartache, divorce, and an old age spent scrounging for meals from trash cans. I can derail that train-of-thought wreck. I don't even have to board it.

"I'm here now," I say, warmly. "It's great that you still have the job. But it's pretty stressful there. Maybe it's time to think about retiring. Do you want to do that? Should we talk about how we could do that?"

Jack shoots me a look mixed with gratitude and surprise, and softly hums a few bars of the *Twilight Zone* theme song.

More than a century ago, the psychologist William James under-stood the link between good-quality attention and self-control, that sine qua non of success and happiness. The trouble, as he saw it then, was that the capacity for attention was fixed, so that "no one who is without it naturally can by any amount of drill or discipline attain it in a very high degree."

But could James have been wrong? Because later that same day, the miracle happens again. While walking with Jack and the kids near one of the reservoirs near our house, Buzz says something provocative, and I say something reactive. Buzz turns to Jack in triumph, saying, "She's just trying to stir things up, because that's how she is."

Am NOT trying, I think. But instead of saying it, and however not-on-task it might seem, I put my arms around Buzz and hug him. It's a lesson I've been learning all this year, but I think I've just made some extra progress.

"You look great in that sweater," I say, meaning it. Then I add, "I love you, Buzz."

I smile at him, and, almost as if he can't help himself, he smiles back. A really stunning smile.

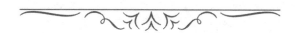

HOW ABOUT
REFRAMABLE?

CHAPTER 10

THE WHITE
CONTENDER

Buddhism is an evolutionary sport.

ROBERT THURMAN

THE CELEBRACION BRIDAL AND TUX SHOP IN DOWNTOWN SAN
Rafael is so crowded with racks of bright silk and polyester brides-
maids' and *quinceañera* gowns that there is hardly room to walk
around. Buzz found the store last month on the Internet, where
he also picked out a white, single-breasted, pin-striped ensemble
that goes by the name of "The White Contender." It comes with a
matching black vest and shirt, a Windsor tie, and shiny white
shoes.

Cedric, the store owner, bustles out from a room in the back,
carrying the suit, still wrapped in plastic, in a boys' size 12. He leads
Buzz to a small dressing room behind a wall pinned with tiny, white
baptismal outfits. At every other bar mitzvah I've been to, the boys
have worn respectable, sober, dark suits. It's only my son who wants
to look like Al Pacino in *Scarface*.

After a few minutes, Buzz calls me into the dressing room, where
Cedric is finishing tying his tie. His eyes are gleaming as he checks
himself out in the full-length mirror, and standing behind him, I'm
pleased to catch the serene expression on my own face.

It's four days before the bar mitzvah ceremony. As late as just a few weeks ago, "The White Contender" was out of the question. Both my father and my sister had urged me in no uncertain terms not to give in, warning that if I didn't, I'd both embarrass our family and spoil Buzz for good. I was dutifully prepared to dig in my heels and tell Buzz that his behavior would reflect on other people, and there are limits, and what about his values, and under no circumstances, and yada yada. Yet as I near the end of this year of bird-dogging all the fruitless ways I've been reacting to the sort of tests Buzz is so skilled at presenting, I've adopted the habit of asking myself a simple question: What would the Dalai Lama do?

And, frankly, I don't think he'd lose much sleep over the white, pin-striped tux. I mean, he might even get a kick out of it. He does seem to have sense of humor. . . .

WHEN I FIRST BEGAN researching this book, I had a grand plan involving Tenzin Gyatso, the fourteenth Dalai Lama of Tibet. I'd imagined taking Buzz to meet him, convinced that even a few moments in the presence of such a master of focus and compassion would inspire and improve my son. We'd have had to fly to Dharamsala, India, of course, where the Dalai Lama has lived for the half century since he fled China's invasion of his homeland. But after all the money and time I'd spent by then on tests and therapies, it didn't seem like such an unreasonable expense.

And so I pursued the goal, sending e-mails and letters beseeching every contact I could think of from my years of reporting on neuroscience and meditation. Apparently, however, that trick about visualizing your dreams isn't always reliable, or maybe I just wasn't doing it right, because the Dalai Lama's monk assistant sent back e-mails brushing me off. I figured I'd better do the next best thing, which was to take Buzz to see His Holiness in Seattle, amid a crowd of fifty thousand, at an April 2008 conference with the timely theme of nurturing compassion in children.

I think back to that day as I watch Buzz turn this way and that in the Celebracion dressing room, while I restrain my urge to pester him to hurry up and get back into his T-shirt and jeans. There's no big rush. True, I've left Max alone back home, but he seemed happy enough, engrossed in a *SpongeBob* episode, and he knows he can call me on the cell phone.

I appear to be moving more deliberately these days, unfamiliar as that feels. What a contrast with last April, before all the neurofeedback and meditation and reflection. Back then, in what was still my customary style, I figured I'd save time and money by flying in and out of Seattle the same day—"parachuting," in the vernacular of foreign correspondents. Buzz didn't seem to mind the rush, thrilled, as usual, to miss school for any reason at all. He set his alarm for 4:15 A.M. and was dressed and ready at the door in fifteen minutes.

Outside it was still dark, the air cool and fresh. I watched Buzz settle joyfully into the backseat of the taxi as we sped away from home. He was wearing his favorite shirt, the shiny, neon-blue Nike number that looks like it came from the Starship *Enterprise*.

Were I to be transported back to that morning as the at-least-somewhat more patient person I've since become, I might have been content to wait until we actually saw the Dalai Lama for Buzz to start making the most of his experience. Back then, I couldn't restrain myself. "Buzz," I said, in my teachable-moment voice, "you know how I went to that meeting at our synagogue a few months ago about preparing for the bar mitzvah? One thing they said is that this is a really sacred year—"

"Mom, you've said that so many times," he groaned.

"Okay, but I'm just saying—"

But then I paused. I could tell what Buzz expected me to say next, having unfortunately heard it so many times before. That I feared he still had lots of room for spiritual growth. That I blamed myself for raising him in self-indulgent Marin County. That I worried that, perhaps as some by-product of his attention issues, he might be missing a moral compass, especially considering he still hadn't gotten started on his philanthropic "mitzvah project" and had asked me just last week what kinds of jobs pay most for the least work.

Chastened, I tried a different tack. "So what do you know about the Dalai Lama?" I asked, brightly.

"Can I get a power-sized Jamba Juice at the airport?" he asked.

IN THE DRESSING ROOM, Buzz sits on a stool to try on the special white silk socks that come with the white shoes. He's taking forever, as he usually does when putting on shoes, but this time I smile to notice him smiling to himself as he fingers the material. I take a deep breath and walk back over to lean on the glass counter next to the cash register, aimlessly studying the array of rhinestone tiaras below my elbows.

I truly hope that if the Dalai Lama ever reads this, he won't mind the audacity of my trying to imagine how he'd react if he were ever, say, reborn as a distracted mom, shouting at her children on a California highway. Based on everything I've read, I'm trusting he'll cut me some slack in consideration for how hard I've worked to be guided by his teachings: to improve my focus, surrender my ego, nurture compassion, and not sweat the small stuff, like the tux.

I wonder if he'd even be somewhat flattered by how much it has helped me to remind myself how *he'd* never yell or curse, even if he were to, say, catch Buzz hitting Max over the head with a soda can, or stealing His Holiness's iPod and loading it with obscene hip-hop tunes. I can't see him ever taking it personally if Buzz called him, for instance, a "butt crack." He'd surely recognize that sort of outburst as simply a variation of human suffering, and meet it with tranquility.

Equanimity can only take me so far, here, of course. As a parent, I'm also obligated to act—to set limits, arrange for consequences (beyond karma), and to offer help when I can. And this brings me to the question of what the Dalai Lama might do about Ritalin.

I've thought a lot about this particular issue over the past year, since despite all my worries about side effects and hopes for alternative treatments, I'm not willing to rule out meds, should Buzz ever need them again. The Buddha himself, after all, advocated the "middle way" of avoiding extremes, particularly the extreme of asceticism, which he called "painful, unworthy, and unprofitable." And how could it not be ascetic, 2,500 years later, to persist in suffering when medication offers relief? The Dalai Lama's brother, Tenzin Choegyal, seems to share this view; I've read that he takes lithium for his bipolar disorder.

I'd hoped to ask the Dalai Lama himself where he stood on this question. But once I realized I wasn't going to get that private audience, I asked Cliff Saron instead. My neuroscientist friend has met with the Dalai Lama several times in recent years and says he has heard him answer similar questions. He assured me, in an e-mail, that His Holiness wouldn't be dogmatic about the meds, since he's never dogmatic about anything. Instead, Saron suggested he'd answer my question with more questions. "What's the motivation? What are the benefits? What are the costs?" Saron wrote, channeling the Tibetan sage.

The middle way in this case, Saron concluded, lies between two difficult truths: "Drugs are not enough without a deep context of self-knowledge and the loving holding of society for an individual's needs. And all the love and care in the world is unlikely to fix a leaky synapse."

So I'm guessing the Dalai Lama wouldn't take either side in the Ritalin Wars. And I'm certain he wouldn't waste time, as I have, in worrying about it.

"If the situation is such that you can do something about it, then there is no need to worry," he has famously said. "If it's not fixable, then there is no help in worrying."

LOOKING BACK, it's embarrassing to remember how much I worried on that day that Buzz and I spent in Seattle. Running late, as usual, I clenched my teeth as we sat in our taxi, stuck in the traffic circling the Bank of America sports arena, where Tenzin Gyatso was scheduled to

appear within the next ten minutes. Of course, of course, we should
have flown in last night, and not cut things this close. Like I always do.

At the airport, the turbaned cabbie had assured us that he knew
the way. But then he'd gotten lost, and I'd had to call Jack, at work,
to look up the directions on the Internet.

Cops were out in force, motioning the cars to keep moving. The
driver in front of us pulled over anyway, to let out his passengers, and
I urged our cabbie to do the same.

"C'mon, you can do it!" I hissed. "Look at that car!"

"Mom!" Buzz scolded. "He's afraid he'll get in trouble with the
police!"

We edged up four more blocks until he finally let us out, and we ran
back together to the arena. But the young guards at the entrance
stopped us, saying I could take my purse inside, but not Buzz's backpack. How arbitrarily nuts was that? There wasn't even a metal de-
tector. So by keeping the backpacks, they were going to outwit
terrorists? I started arguing, even as I knew I was wasting my time.

"Mom, just leave it here," Buzz urged me. "It'll be okay."

I sighed and nodded, and we hurried inside, climbing into the
stands. And there he was already, wearing a bright red robe and
oddly sportive red baseball cap, sitting next to the Reverend Des-
mond Tutu, in a deep pink gown. The image was projected on a giant
screen behind them, affording a close-up view of the thick, dark eyebrows, the shaved head, and the yellow-tinted glasses. The two old
men, friends from way back, sprawled on their chairs, occasionally
chuckling together, as if having a private chat in front of tens of
thousands.

We got there just in time to hear His Holiness say it's a universal
responsibility to feel other people's suffering just as we feel our
own. "Love and compassion are necessities, not luxuries," he told the
packed stadium audience. "When you take care of others, it benefits
you. Others are the ultimate source of our happiness."

At this, Buzz took a bag of potato chips out of his pocket and
started to eat them, with obvious enjoyment. Yet he seemed also
to be listening, even joining in, a few minutes later, in singing the

conference anthem: "We are the seeds of compassion! We're ready to sow the seeds of compassion, right now!"

He sang, but I hung back. Still four months away, back then, from getting my minor in Enlightenment at Spirit Rock, I was hit by a wave of irritation that I was powerless to fend off. For all my admiration of the Dalai Lama, it bugged me how everyone around us was sighing and nodding at his simplest platitudes. Especially the gray-haired woman in the tie-dyed T-shirt, sitting in front of us, who alternated her sighs and applause with turning around and glaring nastily at Buzz, each time he crunched on a potato chip.

Then, right on the heels of my anger, came sadness, as I focused on the half dozen Youth Representatives on stage behind the Dalai Lama. Nominated from local schools, they were all about Buzz's age, but so remarkably poised and earnest, the kind of kids I always used to imagine I'd have: openhearted, expressive, helpful at home, getting perfect grades, playing the flute, and planning meal drives for the homeless. Kids who wouldn't in a thousand reincarnations even dream of calling their own mother a bitch.

Thinking back to that moment, while waiting in the tux shop, I marvel at my unfairness. After all, as a child myself, I wasn't ever like that. Sure, I played the flute and got good grades, but I was also secretive and rebellious, keeping my parents up at night with continually outrageous behavior. How did I come to expect Buzz to be different? And while I'm at it, how come I'm only now really noticing and appreciating his compassion for the cabbie and his patience with the guards—not to mention the way he insisted, before we left the city, that we buy a stuffed animal to bring home to Max?

In the Seattle stadium, however, I was still thinking only: *What am I doing wrong?*

As the conference continued, one of the earnest Youth Representatives asked the Dalai Lama how he had first learned about compassion. He answered as he always does. "Everybody's real teacher of compassion is one's own mother," he said. "There's no doubt."

I jabbed Buzz in the ribs to make sure he registered this. Yet to myself, I was wondering, once again, why something that sounds so

easy would ever be so hard. Teach my own children compassion?
Like the Dalai Lama says, that's what mothers do! The trick, however, is not to cram their little heads with talking points, but to model
the behavior. And, man, there is so much that can get in the way. Like
genes. And inefficient neurotransmitters. And overaroused brain
waves. And the kind of history that could make me react to my child,
so unfairly, as if he were someone else—like, oh, just for instance,
my father.

MY DAD, as I've come to realize only in recent years, was my family
of origin's automatic bad guy, just as Buzz has been in ours. My father
disappointed us so often that it easily obscured the memories of all
the times he was heroically hardworking, loyal, and loving. There was
that day, about thirteen years ago, for instance, after I'd flown back
home from Rio, like a tortoise, to give birth. My parents had shown
up at the hospital just in time to hear me screaming in remorse about
having turned down that epidural. The rest of Buzz's delivery went
smoothly, yet the next day, as Jack and I left the hospital with our
new infant, we discovered that our rental car, parked in the garage,
had been sideswiped. Some Good Samaritan had left a note tucked
behind the windshield wiper: "Green BMW hit your car!" it read,
along with my father's license-plate number.

Clearly my father had parked next to us while visiting and either
didn't see what he'd done, or let it slip his mind. I never assumed he
meant it personally, or even that he'd recognized the car. Nonetheless, for many years, "Green BMW Hit Your Car" was my private
motto for all the times he'd hurt me or my siblings, intentionally
or not.

Then came this year of trying to see life through my son's eyes—a
year in which I found myself repeatedly distracted by thoughts of my
father. Realizing that I needed to better understand our family history, I interviewed friends and relatives back in Minneapolis, and
then questioned my parents, piecing together more of the circumstances surrounding the pivotal event of my father's decision to move

west in 1961. It wasn't, after all, really the jaunty adventure they'd often painted it to be when I was growing up. At the time, my father's career options had narrowed. He'd clashed with the administration at the Jewish hospital where he was chief of the ear, nose, and throat department, by siding with a family that had sued the hospital for malpractice after a horrific accident, when their child was left with brain damage after what should have been a routine operation. When he tried to switch to a different employer, a Christian hospital in what was then a fiercely anti-Semitic city, he was told that they'd already filled their quota of Jews.

If it was difficult, as my father has since told me, to ignore his own father's pleas for him to stay put, it must have been wrenching after his mother died of a stroke that same year. But in fact, my father's troubles were just starting. On his first drive out west, to meet his new office partners, he contracted a lung disease known as "valley fever," which his own doctor initially misdiagnosed as lung cancer. My dad spent his first year at his new job coughing and feverish, heading to bed as soon as he got home, fearing he wouldn't survive.

Hindsight has revealed for me the similarities between that hard year for my parents and the year I spent waiting to have brain surgery: a year in which, as I've only recently come to understand, I lost a connection with Buzz that has taken a year of determined attention to restore. In addition to the challenges of work, children, and illness, I was coping—much like my father—with an undiagnosed mental disorder. And despite my best intentions, some damage was done. Unlike my parents, however, who struggled with their hardships in an era of tremendous stigma about mental health, I've been able to rely on psychotherapists, primarily including Dr. Y., in addition to medication, meditation, and neurofeedback. Along the way, I've come to appreciate that even as my mother urged me to "Understand your father!" after yet another night when he had chased one of my brothers through the house with his belt, she couldn't—through no fault of her own—have begun to tell me how.

What would the Dalai Lama tell me to do about my dad? Surely, he'd urge me to investigate my attachment to those negative memories, such as the green BMW, and to consider the things my father did that never got as much attention. Like the way he labored so patiently for so many years, performing surgeries and cleaning sinuses, to put me and my siblings through college. Or the hilarious, bawdy limericks he wrote for every significant family occasion, and how touchingly and vainly he'd try, each year, to escape from the torment of sitting through a day of Yom Kippur services by suggesting we take a family drive to see the fall foliage. Or, in particular, how he was the only one I knew who was willing to accompany me to the gruesome slide show my brain surgeon somehow thought would help prepare me for the operation. With a certain lack of empathy for his audience, the surgeon took pride in showing off some of his particularly harrowing cases. My father held my hand throughout the presentation, stage-whispering, "*Yours* isn't going to be anything like that!"

Now that he's eighty-five years old, my father has been making more of a conscious effort to slow down and listen to me and my siblings. He still frequently behaves badly, with the difference that he now usually ends up apologizing, sometimes even acknowledging that he can be rash and insensitive. It's all part of what he calls "cramming for the finals."

I wish he hadn't been so angry so often when I was growing up. I wish he'd been able to get the help he needed. I wish I could have helped him, or even understood him better. I can't do anything now about any of that. There's one thing I can do, however. There've been times, recently, when my father has felt particularly misunderstood and has told me, "I wish I had a friend like me."

And I've answered: "You do. It's me."

IN THE TUX SHOP, my cell phone rings. It's Max.

"When are you coming hooooome?" he asks, eliciting yet another twinge of guilt about all the extra time I've been spending with his brother.

"We're on our way, sweetie! Just another fifteen minutes!" I tell him. My voice is bright and warm, as I put into practice the best thing I learned from the Dalai Lama in Seattle. Someone asked him, as people often do, how he is able to remain so peaceful and positive, given all the world's problems and suffering.

"You pay attention to the arising of emotions, and know what is the best emotion under the circumstances," he answered. "To reduce one emotion, one must cultivate a counterforce."

Like so much of what the Dalai Lama says, this at first sounded so simple. Yet it went to the heart of my struggle, this past year, to replace anger with equanimity, judgment with insight and compassion.

As I've gradually come to understand, the main trouble with impulsive, distracted people is that we so naturally tend to invite anger and judgment. Civilization depends on trust, but our lapses violate it. We provoke and pester, cause conflicts and may even hurt others, usually unintentionally and frequently against our best interests.

For a parent, however, responding instinctively—angrily, judgmentally—is always destructive. You join a chain reaction, trading negative for negative, as the conflicts escalate, like road rage. I've come to believe that the only way to break this chain is to keep in mind William James's idea that what you pay attention to becomes your reality and, whenever possible, to keep my focus fixed on the best parts of people's natures. There's a bright side, too, to today's otherwise oppressive hailstorm of data about mental disorders—from attention deficit to oppositional defiant, to bipolar to Asperger's. If we're patient, and lucky, and do our best, perhaps all of our confused debate about character-vs.-disorder and explanation-vs.-excuse may one day lead us to a new era of understanding.

Buzz pops out of the dressing room, back in his street clothes. Cedric smiles as he hands me the bill, and I take out my checkbook, focusing on trying to substitute gratitude for all I've learned in place of the panic threatening to emerge at the thought of all the other checks I'll be writing in the next four days—the caterer, the florist, the band . . . After all, I've dodged one little bullet. On our first trip here, Buzz lingered for several minutes over a picture of a "zoot" tux with a long jacket, as Cedric eagerly asked if he wanted to see the hat and chain that came with it.

I'm grateful that he didn't, but I'm grateful, too, for the way Rabbi Michael responded when I finally took my father's suggestion, last week, and asked what the rabbi thought of Buzz wearing a white tux as he becomes a bar mitzvah.

"Yasher koach!" he promptly said, using the Hebrew phrase for "more power to him!" It's Buzz's day, after all. And in the years to come, I can only hope he'll find more friends and allies and authority figures to say *"Yasher koach!"* to his wild ideas. In the meantime, I'm going to keep practicing shifting my attention—deliberately, now, and again and again, like a fan at a tennis match—appreciating how my particular son has been teaching me the basics of compassion, in ways I might never have learned them as the mother of an easier kid.

CHAPTER 11

KNOTS TO UNDO

Shake and shake the ketchup bottle.
None will come out, and then a lot'l.

OGDEN NASH

"MOM, DO YOU HAVE THE COPY OF MY HAFTARAH PORTION?"

The synagogue is filled. The guests are already seated. The start of the service is minutes away. *Did anyone tell me I was supposed to bring the haftarah portion?*

I remembered the checks for the band and the caterer. I remembered the list of people the photographer couldn't forget to shoot. I remembered the copy of my blessing for Buzz, and remembered to remind Jack to bring his. *But nobody ever told me about the freaking haftarah portion! And now I'm going to sabotage my own son's bar mitzvah!*

By sheer coincidence, it's "National AD/HD Awareness Week."

Over the past three days:

I drove over the curb at the synagogue while the kids were distracting me by fighting, and popped a brand-new tire.

Lehman Brothers went bankrupt, leading to a historic plunge in the Dow of nine hundred points over just two days.

New York magazine ran a story about troubles in the book publishing industry—my current employer—titling it, "The End."

Aside from these worries, this feels a lot like the day Jack and I got married. I've got the same internally carbonated feeling. Part of me wants this to go on forever, even as there's also this other little part that wants it to be over already. So many things could still go wrong. . . .

Buzz is a vision in "The White Contender," looking vaguely like John Travolta in *Saturday Night Fever*. As I've anxiously reminded him more than once this past week, those fancy clothes will only make it worse if he's not prepared, risking a fiasco that will live on in the memories of the most important people in our lives. The crowd in the synagogue includes not only Buzz's best friend and a half dozen other kids from school, but my parents, three siblings (from as far away as Massachusetts), three siblings-in-law, six nieces and nephews, eight members of my writers' group, and several friends, including Sarah (the mother of Commando Demando), Phil and Sally, and even Cliff Saron.

While I remain stunned by Buzz's unexpected question, Rabbi Michael darts off without a word and then materializes again, with a copy of the haftarah portion. Usually, Rabbi Michael exudes tranquillity, cracking jokes and grinning away. Today he's all business: leaning forward, dark eyes intent behind thick glasses. He leads my parents, Jack, Buzz, Max, and me, up a short flight of stairs behind the synagogue to his office for a brief, private blessing.

"Can we take pictures?" Jack asks.

"Just in here," he says, tapping his forehead.

We stand together in the small room, where he tells us to put our arms around one another. Buzz is by my side, as I look straight into my father's eyes. *They're full of tears!* My mother has been crying nonstop ever since she walked into the synagogue, but that's what she does at all significant occasions. My father doesn't cry, at least not that I've ever seen before. I'm betting that he's thinking what most of the rest of us are thinking, something like Damn, *how time flies!*

As if reading my mind, Rabbi Michael looks from face to face and warns us: "You're going to blink and at twelve-fifteen it will be over. Keep your eyes open."

The ritual prayer shawl, the tallis, that Buzz will wear today was sewn half a century ago by Jack's grandmother Hannah, a Ukrainian immigrant, when Jack became a bar mitzvah. It has knotted fringes, called *tzitzit,* on all four corners: eye-catching reminders to keep the commandments.

"Hannah is with us today," Rabbi Michael is saying. "And so are all of our ancestors back to Mount Sinai."

He then turns to Buzz and tells him how proud all of us are of his hard work, how much we treasure his extraordinary spirit, and how great he looks in that tux. Then he recites the blessing over the tallis and shows Buzz how to envelope himself in it.

Buzz hasn't once stopped grinning; I've never seen him so proud. Rabbi Michael leads him to the bimah, while Jack, Max, and I take our seats in the front row. I hear my young nephew, David, coughing hoarsely a few rows back. Three days from now, both Max and Jack will come down with pneumonia.

Buzz stands behind the pulpit like he owns it, right under the *ner tamid,* the "eternal light" meant to symbolize God's constant presence. He takes a deep breath, composing himself, and commences to lead the congregation in the first of the Hebrew blessings, the Sh'ma: "Hear O Israel, the Lord our God, the Lord is one. . . ."

His voice is a little scratchy, but he seems confident, even as if he's enjoying himself. Cantor David is standing nearby, ready to help, but smiling to see there's no need. I mouth the words along with him, praying with all my agnostic heart.

Rabbi Michael asks if anyone has any miracles they'd like to mention. Jack's brother, Jerry, a symphony violist in an elegant Italian suit, wisecracks: "Jack's wearing a tie!" Someone else says she's grateful her husband's CAT scan came back clear. I know I should probably say something—thank all the people who came, perhaps—but

I don't trust my voice. Plus, the time for gratitude will be when this is over. Assuming Buzz doesn't make good on his threat, as of just yesterday, to yell, "God bless America!" at the end, or make that crack about George Bush that we edited out of his speech, or demonstrate in front of the entire congregation how very little he has been studying.

YOU MIGHT THINK I could stay focused and present for my own son's bar mitzvah ceremony, which I've looked forward to now for more than a year. But even now, my mind starts to wander, and before I know it, I'm once again lost in the past, revisiting the terrible, obligatory parent-and-child pre–bar mitzvah retreat I ended up at with Buzz last spring, at a woodsy Jewish camp in Santa Rosa.

"The parents go, too?" my mother said. "How nice! We never did that when you were growing up."

"The parents have to go?" my friend Susan, from my writers' group, said. *What are they thinking?*

Buzz had fought for weeks against going, as I dug in my heels. *Why can't we be the kind of family for whom this kind of thing is a piece of cake?* Instead, we were still squabbling even an hour after arriving that first night, as soon as Buzz took one look around the hall filled with kids who were ignoring him, and at the dinner of paprika-speckled rubbery chicken and withered green beans, and tearfully demanded that we leave.

"Look," I said desperately. "Let's negotiate."

"I don't negotiate with terrorists!" he wailed.

I ended up getting him to go to the evening service and meetings that night with the promise that we'd sneak out for breakfast, just the two of us, the next morning.

"If we sleep in the car, we'll be all ready to go!" he said.

"Don't be silly," I retorted. But that was where I found him at dawn the next morning: in his sleeping bag, reading a Rick Riordan novel with a flashlight. I'd spent a nearly sleepless night myself, on a stinky mattress in a room with five other moms I wasn't friends with and who were at least as miserable as I was about being there.

Our breakfast was nice, though—at least right up until the huge tantrum Buzz threw when I insisted we go back for the rest of the day's program. Back then I was angry and disappointed. But here in the synagogue, I wonder if the Dalai Lama would ever have gone on that retreat, or if he might easily have recognized that it wasn't ever really necessary—that, after all, our attendance had no bearing whatsoever on the magic of this moment, and the flawless job my exceptionally well-behaved son is doing up there—

SQUAWWWKKK!

A burst of static interrupts Buzz's chanting. Several members of the congregation wince, but Buzz takes it in stride, with a suave smile, a pause, and another deliberate inhale.

SQUAWK-SQUEEREEEKKK!

Cantor David hustles backstage to fiddle with the sound system, which squawks twice more before he's done. *What bad luck! How could this not wreck anyone's composure!* I recognize a subtle change in Buzz's expression—a Daniel Craig–like flash of muted outrage—but then he catches my eye and responds to what he must have seen as my unsubtle alarm by raising two fingers in a peace sign.

We have to stand for the next prayer, which draws my attention to my trembling knees. This ceremony may be all about loosening the tie between a child and his mother, but I've never, since those first blissful months of his babyhood, felt more joyfully connected to him.

The joy lasts barely a minute, however, before Max, who can only take so much of his brother's glory, starts making loud chomping noises, imploding the air inside his mouth. Buzz shoots us a dark look, as Jack puts his hand over Max's mouth, and Max bites Jack's fingers, while I hear snickers from members of my writers' group, seated just behind us.

Now, at last, Rabbi Michael brings out the Torah, and begins the part of the service in which family members are called to chant blessings before and after Buzz reads. Max quiets down, and in what seems like a very short time, we're ready for Buzz's *d'var Torah,* his speech to interpret the reading.

Jack and I have taken seats to the left of the ark, the ornate cabinet containing the Torah. Max sits by himself for half a minute in the front row, but then can't control himself any longer and crawls on all fours across the short space of carpet to sit with us. People giggle, and I wrap my arm around him for a hug. *Just get us through the next hour.*

I've known for the past three weeks what Buzz is going to say, but it still strikes me as wondrous. He has chosen, all by himself, to talk about "patience and perseverance." Which means he has either been actually listening to me, or understands what I've most hoped to teach him.

It's not a bad speech, and Buzz reads it well, with good pacing and eye contact. He talks about the patience of his immigrant ancestors, and the Israelites wandering their way to the Promised Land, and then elaborates, with a characteristic flourish, about how the emperor penguin walks up to one hundred miles through blizzards en route to its breeding ground, "while the cheetah must wait until the perfect moment to sprint up to seventy miles to catch food, or starve!"

He cites Mahatma Gandhi's long campaign of civil disobedience, and Barack Obama's perseverance in the nineteen-month primary season finally nearing its end. He doesn't say anything rude about Bush, merely noting how a lack of patience helped get us into the Iraq War. And then comes my favorite part, in which Buzz tells the congregation how he still remembers the patience of his first babysitter, Alzira, back when he was a toddler in Rio, and how he plans to send her a portion of his gifts. (I'd had to talk him out of putting a sign up in the synagogue lobby to this effect.) Despite my worries that he'd never stop to think about anyone else this year, Buzz had come up with the Alzira project all by himself, after overhearing Jack and me worrying about how she was doing.

"As I become a man today according to our tradition, I know I still need to work on being more patient in my own life, with my parents, my brother, my friends, and my homework," Buzz says, nearing the finish line. "I hope I can do so with the humility of Moses, who even as he knew he'd never reach the Promised Land himself, blessed the people before he died."

Jack and I exchange a wide-eyed look. The scariest part is over. Our son has come through this with grace, and he knows it. This achievement will be part of his life story, something he'll always re-member.

I stand in front of Buzz and read my blessing to him.

I tell him that he has given himself the best possible blessing. That he has such a strong will and is going to go so far, *if he can just learn* when to hold himself back. But then I catch his eyes as they're rising to the ceiling. *I can't stop nagging him, even now!*

I suck in my breath. I've been told over and over again in recent months, to the point where I've had to believe it, that I'm overly anxious. And although Buzz has indisputably needed me to worry about him through this past year, it's suddenly clear, even to me, that he is no longer the flailing boy I made my personal and profes-sional project. He's now someone else: a young man who can wear a white tux with panache. So now I must change, too. While I have no illusions (and time will soon enough prove me right) that this fairytale scene means my mothering heartaches are all in the past, I know that to the extent that he keeps making progress, it's my duty to step back. On the one hand, I should strive to be a con-stant, loving presence in the background—like the *ner tamid.* Yet I'll have to find another mooring for my free-floating worries, an-other source of electricity, another life's mission. *What the heck will ever measure up?*

Maybe nothing will again. But for now, I simply take a literal step back from my son, skipping over most of the rest of what I'd planned to say. I tell him *mazel tov,* and that I love him, and I can't wait to see what he comes up with next.

And then it's Jack's turn.

His message is graceful, funny, and diplomatic. He gives his own nod to Buzz's strong drive, recalling how, as a ten-month-old baby tasting ice cream for the first time, Buzz yanked back the spoon from Jack's hand "with alarming force." But then Jack talks of his capacity for sweetness, how extraordinarily kind he is to younger children (barring Max, of course, but Jack leaves that part out), and ends up with a blessing that fits in the names of each of the close family members in the room.

Rabbi Michael is now standing in front of Buzz, telling him, "You not only chanted Hebrew from the depths of your *kishkes,* but you also made us see what it means to be an active citizen in the world. All that light inside you is an inspiration. Bring it back out to the universe. We ask God that you know patience and perseverance."

"Thanks," Buzz whispers, smiling away.

He swirls around to give Max a high-five. *Party time!*

We've hired the Red Hot Chachkas klezmer band, the same group that played at the Hanukah party where I had that fight with Phil. The bandleader, Julie, pesters everyone to dance, and I weave around the room hugging and getting hugged. Buzz, Jack, and Max get lifted up in chairs, just like in the movies, and when it gets to my turn, the members of my writers' group rush in to raise me up, pretty much as they've done for the past two years. The room whips around, and the rest of the afternoon whips by.

Toward evening, my parents and brothers and sister and in-laws crowd into our living room, nibbling at leftovers, while Buzz and his young cousins and guests trash our bedroom. Within the next two hours, there will be owies, recriminations, and a bitter dispute over a broken Xbox game. Right now we're just marveling over how well Buzz did.

"Maybe we underestimated that kid," my dad is saying.

In the kitchen, I catch sight of Buzz taking a plate of lox out of the refrigerator. Jack sees him, too, and says, resignedly, "There goes my lox."

Buzz turns around and looks back at us. "I'm going to leave some for Dad," he announces just before running back to the bedroom, "because being a man means you make good decisions."

"OMG," I say.

"Hey, maybe the bar mitzvah was worth it," Jack says.

I'M ENDING THIS HERE, while it's still this good. There've been some awful bumps in the road so far, and I don't need a team of neuropsychologists to tell me that more bumps are in store. On the other hand, I know we've made some good progress. I no longer worry, for instance, that Buzz is going to end up in jail.

Still, this by no means suggests I don't worry about other things. I recognize the heightened risk that Buzz could die ignobly, as the result of some impulsive move—like so many I've made myself—in which case, for the rest of my life, I'll be a bad parent. Or he could die at the end of a brilliant life, in which case I'll be a genius. Either way, eventually, global warming will get us, or maybe an asteroid, or cancer from bisphenol-whatsis, or a North Korean nuke. Or something more humdrum, like old age, or a car crash. All we can really count on is having our lives end up like those intricate sandpaintings that Tibetan monks spend hours upon hours on to make perfect, and then blow away. Which nonetheless leaves us with the choice of what we'll do about our lives right now.

I've asked Buzz several times throughout this year if he wanted to read what I've written, yet he has always turned me down. "Too boring!" he said the other day, when I pressed him for a reason.

"Okay, well, what if you just write something for the end?" I proposed. "Even something small! Even a paragraph!"

"How much would you pay for that?" he asked. "I mean, for a professional contribution like that, I'm thinking $1,000."

"I'm thinking more like $50, at most, and only if it's worth it," I said. "But what would you write, if you wrote something?"

He mumbled something I couldn't hear.

"Huh?"

"Keep trying!"

"Keep trying?"

"Yeah, keep trying!"

It works for me.

WHAT ELSE WORKED

At the end of this year of researching ways to make life calmer and happier for my family, I have to acknowledge that no single approach topped the decision to collaborate with my son on this book. From that moment, not only was I free to devote extra time to our problem, but a source of frustration and shame—*the trouble with Buzz*—became a (mostly) mutually beneficial project. Looking at my son—and my own hitherto perplexing history—with my investigative reporter's eye afforded me a different perspective I hadn't known I needed. I was able to listen more dispassionately, and more effectively, and finally to appreciate how much I needed to cope with my own distraction before I could help Buzz with his. Conscious of the rare privilege of this experience, I can only hope that some of what I've learned may help other parents in my overloaded boat.

The über-lesson is that there's no silver bullet—no pill, or herb, or exercise—that is going to "cure" your child. That said, in my opinion, some widely recommended strategies are clearly more helpful than others, while some should be avoided altogether.

Meds and Neurofeedback

As I've described, I gradually came to accept that some medications can help some children so dramatically that, despite the many drawbacks, and until something more effective shows up, I wouldn't rule them out as an option. At the same time, my research and personal experience has made me a particular fan of neurofeedback, which under ideal circumstances is much safer than medication, and may be more long-lasting, despite the drawbacks of how much time and money it requires. Stay tuned for the pilot results of the first major federal study of this practice, expected in 2011. In the meantime, a growing amount of anecdotal evidence—including my own—is encouraging. With the help of more than thirty neurofeedback sessions with a skilled practitioner, I considerably lowered my baseline level of anxiety, which appears to have had a good effect on everyone around me, particularly Buzz. Buzz had a similar number of sessions, which seemed to help so much that he was able to forgo medication for nearly a year. Toward the end of eighth grade, however, he ran into such serious trouble in school, and once again seemed so angry and unhappy, that I offered him a choice: more neurofeedback or meds. He opted for the meds, but this time we got a prescription for a shorter-acting stimulant formula and also took Buzz in for an EKG, to screen for preexisting heart conditions, as recommended by the American Heart Association. While he took the pills, from May to July of 2009, Buzz's behavior and mood improved dramatically, as it did when he took meds in seventh grade. The catch this time was that he suffered from terrible insomnia, so much that, in the month I'm writing this, he quit the medication once again. We're currently investigating non-stimulant formulas and discussing whether to try more neurofeedback. It's still a work in progress. Even so, I've been encouraged that Buzz has come to understand and accept the basic idea that he needs help, and that help is available, even though it may not be ideal. It's a level of self-awareness that I can only wish more people enjoyed.

Supplements

Max's skepticism in the opening pages of this book aside, there's credible research indicating that fish oil—or more broadly, omega-3 fatty acids, which you can also get from flax seeds or olive oil, and some nuts—can help with attention and moods. Most modern diets are deficient in omega-3s, supplying only about 5 percent of what our ancestors consumed in the 1900s. And that's bad news, considering these essential fats not only help prevent heart disease but also support brain health. Some studies suggest a serious omega-3 deficiency may cause or exacerbate ADD symptoms by interfering with neurotransmitters, including serotonin and dopamine. Experts recommend that children take up to 2.5 grams a day of an omega-3 supplement such as purified fish oil, while adults can take up to 5 grams.

As far as other ballyhooed supplements are concerned, however, it's wise to proceed with caution. This thriving, multibillion-dollar industry remains almost entirely unregulated, and the supplements are usually costly and sometimes unsafe. The Harvard ADD expert Todd Rose recalls how, back in the 1980s, his well-meaning grandmother persuaded his mother to buy a brand of powdered soy shakes that were taken off the market after federal regulators discovered they were contaminated with salmonella bacteria. Several million Americans, meanwhile, take ginkgo biloba and/or ginseng, encouraged by prominent experts who recommend them for problems with attention. Yet studies have shown that ginkgo may interfere with blood clotting, particularly when combined with aspirin, while ginseng has been linked to high blood pressure and rapid heartbeat.

Toxins

Food additives, particularly artificial colors and flavors, as well as benzoate preservative, appear to increase hyperactivity in children, including those without ADD. For pregnant women and children, pesticide exposure is especially risky. Animal studies have linked even low-level contact with the common insecticides known as organophosphates to hyperactive behavior.

Exercise

Regular, strenuous exercise stands out as a particularly helpful strategy for coping with serious distraction. I've been an exercise junkie all my life, but never understood why I was so drawn to it, and so improved by it, until I heard a talk by Dr. John Ratey, who has written a whole book on the subject (*Spark: The Revolutionary New Science of Exercise and the Brain*). Exercise increases blood flow to the brain, while elevating important neurotransmitters such as dopamine and serotonin, and increasing levels of BDNF, or brain-derived neurotrophic factor, a protein that strengthens cells and improves intracellular connections needed for learning. Children who begin an exercise program of just twenty to forty minutes a day have been shown to make significant improvements in "executive functions" such as planning and organizing. As I've mentioned, I've pulled out all the stops to get Buzz involved in regular aerobic activity other than cardio-punching his brother.

Buyer Beware

I ended up avoiding several touted "drug-free" treatments for serious distraction, despite abundant Internet testimonials, usually by people with names like "Sheila G." The tremendous frustration encountered by parents coping with a child's attention deficit disorder—plus the stigma and worries surrounding medication—can make us easy victims for supposed miracle cures. Over the past decade, the U.S. Federal Trade Commission has taken action against several purported treatments making unproven claims, beginning in 1998 with a dietary regime marketed as "God's Recipe." A good rule of thumb is to find a doctor you trust and check with him or her before trying anything adventurous.

While I had little trouble resisting the urge to send in hair samples for analysis, to see if heavy metals were sapping our focus, I did, for a few weeks, consider shelling out $4,970 on the "Dore Method," a heavily advertised approach for learning disorders including attention deficit disorder. I was drawn to it, along with thousands of other parents in the United States and United Kingdom, after reading the enthusiastic endorsement of Edward *"Driven to Distraction"* Hallowell, who at the time was a paid consultant for the company, and who told me in an interview that both his son and wife had benefited from it. The patented technique consists of a series of exercises, to be performed for about ten minutes, twice a day, over the course of a year, including throwing and catching a bean bag and standing on a "balance board"—a wooden disk that wobbles around on a ball. The purported goal of all this activity is to stimulate the cerebellum, a brain region known to be involved in coordination, working memory, attention, and impulse control. The program requires regular appointments to monitor progress, which meant that Buzz and I would have had to make several trips to Los Angeles, the Dore center location nearest to our home.

It seemed worth exploring, until I focused on the part where Buzz would have to keep up with the disciplined exercises. I had only to recall our pitched battles over his refusal to practice the piano, before he quit, to realize what a crazy dream *that* was, and eventually decided that any child capable of completing the year-long program might not have really needed it in the first place. Thus I saved $4,935, plus whatever all those trips to LA would have cost, by instead buying a $35 balance board, which I kept for several months in the hallway between the front door and the kitchen. Buzz has spent a lot of time standing on it, although I have no way of knowing whether that has improved his cerebellum's function.

One apparently promising strategy I haven't yet tried—mostly because I ran out of time and money—is a five-week, computer-based program called Cogmed Working Memory Training, designed by the neuroscientist Torkel Klingberg, based at the prestigious Karolinska Institute in Sweden. Peer-reviewed studies support claims that this type of regimen can help improve working memory, attention, and self-control—the main deficits involved in ADD. In one laboratory project, led by neuroscientist Michael Posner, researchers trained preschool children with a similar five-day computer-based program. The project achieved such success that Posner has publicly called for attention-training to become part of early education. The Cogmed program costs about $2,000 and requires a commitment of up to forty-five minutes a day, for five days a week—a significant disciplinary hurdle, but more doable than the Dore Method. Currently the only way to try the program is through a certified coach.

Meditation

As I've noted, that terrible catch-22 of needing discipline to improve one's discipline certainly also applies to meditation, a fact that is especially discouraging when you consider all the research suggesting that mindfulness training may be particularly helpful for people with attention deficit disorder. Happier news is that some benefits of mindfulness can be achieved without marathons of sitting on a pillow. In recent years, for instance, a Virginia psychologist named Nirbhay Singh has trained hundreds of aggressive children, and their mothers, to shift attention away from angry conflicts with the simple trick of focusing on the soles of their feet. Practicing for just twenty minutes over five days, the former combatants have reportedly gained a new awareness of the relationship between attention and emotion, which in turn has helped them exercise more control. Singh has reported such success that several other therapists throughout the country have begun to copy the simple technique. Meanwhile, mindfulness training is increasingly making its way into U.S. public schools, where creative teachers have been discovering other user-friendly strategies. (Buzz's personal favorite is an exercise in which you slowly and deliberately eat a Hershey's chocolate kiss.)

Education

To my regret, I ended up reporting the chapter on education too late to be able to use what I learned to help spare Buzz most of his exceptionally awful experience between fifth and eighth grade. School is often where clinically distracted kids suffer the most, yet avoiding the pitfalls unfortunately takes a lot more awareness, understanding, and time than most parents have. "Schools bank on parents not understanding the law—they bank on our ignorance," warns Mary Durheim, a McAllen, Texas, educational consultant and past president of the national lobbying group Children and Adults with Attention Deficit/Hyperactivity Disorder.

I didn't know, for instance, until I started digging—because no teacher or school administrator ever volunteered the information—that as a parent of a child with a suspected or confirmed learning disability, including attention deficit disorder, you have a legal right to request, and, if justified, receive, special support from your child's public school. Section 504 of the U.S. Rehabilitation Act of 1973 is the applicable law in most cases. This piece of civil rights legislation prohibits discrimination based on "mental or physical impairment that substantially limits one or more major life activity," including learning, concentrating, and interacting with others. The law says your child must have equal access to education—meaning that if he needs more time on tests, note-taking help, tutoring, or even social skills training to stay in school, the school must provide or pay for it.

Public schools must comply with this law on pain of losing their federal aid. Upon your request, the school district is obligated to give you a copy of its Section 504 policies, including an explanation of how you may appeal its decisions. The law also allows parents to request an evaluation of their child, which in turn may lead to assistance referred to as a "504 plan." Accommodations may include tutoring, counseling, extra time on tests, access to a computer, and an extra set of textbooks to use at home. Active kids may be allowed to sit on "fit balls" or hold squishy toys to control their tendency to fidget. Particularly enlightened school officials may also encourage your child's teacher to devote extra attention to make sure he or she is engaged in the classroom, to employ more frequent praise and encouragement, and to offer special rewards for progress.

For more severe learning problems, another federal law applies: the IDEA, the Individuals with Disabilities Education Act of 2004. Under the IDEA, parents have the right to ask that the school screen their child for a disability, which is potentially a way to avoid paying high fees to a private specialist. Yet if school authorities don't think tests are needed, they can turn you down. Their tests are also much more limited, as a rule, than those offered by the private industry. Children who qualify under this system are eligible for what's known as an individualized education program, or IEP: a rigorous system of accommodations and regular meetings to monitor them. The 504 plan, in contrast, has the advantage of being faster, more flexible, and less stigmatizing.

All that said, it's worth keeping in mind that any progress you make on behalf of your child will ultimately depend on factors including but not limited to school administrators' capacity, enthusiasm, budgets, and how much you're personally willing to educate yourself and others and/or sink time into meetings and bureaucratic appeals.

Out of a combination of initial ignorance, distraction, inertia, and compassion for school officials who seemed all but overwhelmed trying to help kids who were in worse shape than Buzz, I ultimately accepted Buzz's schools' decisions that even though he was getting low grades, working far below his ability, receiving constant reprimands and punishments, and hating school more every day, he wasn't eligible for a formal assistance plan, since he wasn't actually failing. Over the years, however, I nonetheless pestered school officials sufficiently so that he did receive some sporadic extra support, including random visits with a counselor, front-row seating to limit distractions, and an unfortunately named "Special Friends" class in social skills. The first two tactics helped somewhat, yet experts I later interviewed confirmed my suspicion that social skills classes are rarely effective. Students, to be sure, can be trained to recite back instructions about the value of eye contact, sharing, and playing fair, yet that doesn't mean they'll be able to follow them. You also risk having the class turn into a sort of deviancy-training workshop, in which the worst-behaving kids teach the others *their* skills.

Probably the single most effective thing I did for Buzz at school was to provide his seventh-grade teachers with copies of his test results from our neuropsychologist's evaluation. The teachers seemed impressed in particular by the clear finding of the gap between Buzz's high-level verbal skills and his mental processing speed, which encouraged them to stop assuming he was simply not trying.

Meanwhile, the more I learned, as I researched this book, the more I changed the way I talked to Buzz's teachers when they complained—*so often!*—about his behavior. I'd started out, circa second grade, in a chronic cringe, embarrassed by their assumptions about my parenting and quick to apologize. Then I passed through a brief rebellious phase, angry at their readiness to judge him, and me, instead of trying to understand. By Buzz's last year of middle school, however, I'd adopted a new tactic that preserved my self-esteem and occasionally even won some respect. Whenever teachers accused him of bad behavior, I'd hear them out calmly and ask questions to make sure I understood. I'd ask how they thought I could support them, and assure them that that was my intent. But I'd end every session with the same question, which was, "So what is he doing in class that you *like?*" Thus, for instance, a teacher who called to gripe about how Buzz's handwriting looked "like he's *inebriated,*" making her feel as if he didn't care, would recall that he'd enthusiastically participated in that week's current-events quiz—and maybe keep in mind, the next time she saw him, that he wasn't all bad, after all.

AS I COMPLETE THIS BOOK, now nine months after the formal end of our dedicated year, I'm profoundly grateful for the progress that Buzz and I have made. We haven't achieved Nirvana, not by a long shot. I still yell more than I should. Jack still hangs back more than *he* should. Buzz and Max still fight more than I can bear. Even so, the fights have gradually become much less frequent and less hurtful, while I often see the kids playing peacefully together, and looking forward to seeing each other after they've been apart.

Buzz finished his middle school career with a flurry of detentions and an F in algebra. Yet his overall record, teachers' recommendations, and some signs of nascent enthusiasm on his entrance application sufficed to get him accepted at that private school he'd fallen in love with, with an offer of partial financial aid (although we may still have to sell the kidney). At this writing, he plans to enroll in just four weeks, and I'm eager to see if he'll still need medication when he's

taking classes with an 8:1 student/teacher ratio, and when I'm counting on a kinder, gentler social environment to help bring out his best.
And let me just add that in the meantime, I'm also counting on the
Obama administration to fulfill its promise to reform public education, so that similar advantages might one day be available to many
more kids who are now so cruelly and routinely defeated in classrooms all over this country.

In closing, I'm also happy to report that by better monitoring the
way I spend my time—a lesson I learned while reporting the chapter
on chronophages—I've been able to pare down my schedule enough
to keep doing more of what I'd really like to do. Even as my husband
and children at least occasionally confirm my sense that I'm paying
better-quality attention to them, I've found time to, among other
things, adopt a two-year-old poodle mix named Daisy. She had run
away from two previous families but immediately seemed at home in
ours, where she delighted in chasing Buzz around the house, knocking over chairs, and ripping up Max's stuffed animals. Much like
meditation, dog ownership is a superb intervention for clinical distraction, with the similar catch that it's particularly hard for distracted people to find the time for it. Daisy is a walking neurofeedback
machine, encouraging everyone she meets to wag more and bark less.
She also models forgiveness, her own attention span being much too
short to hold a grudge. Buzz has renamed her Dougal (from the dog
in *The Magic Roundabout* TV series) and copies the way she nuzzles
my hand for a scratch behind the ears. At night, she follows me on
my reading rounds, first to Max's room, and then to Buzz's, and finally to join Jack as I squabble with him over sections of the morning's *New York Times.* The other day, Max said, "Daisy is proof that
God is nice." Buzz agreed, and, frankly, I don't care who they've got
in mind—Charlton Heston, Jesus Christ, or the Buddha. I just hope
they keep feeling that way.

San Anselmo, July 2009

NOTES

PROLOGUE

Page 5 *Attention deficit disorder, or ADD*
Perhaps fittingly, American experts have been inconsistent in the manner in which they refer to a flickering state of mind. Throughout this book, for simplicity's sake, I've decided to avoid the cumbersome current formal acronym of AD/HD in favor of the simpler and still-popular ADD. From time to time, I'll also use phrases such as "seriously distracted" or "scatterbrained" to refer to the condition clinically defined, as of this writing, as "attention-deficit/hyperactivity disorder" in the *Diagnostic and Statistical Manual,* the psychiatric industry's atlas. From 1980 to 1987, attention deficit disorder was the formal name for a phenomenon that has had half a dozen other names in its century-old history. (And I've been warned that psychiatrists may come up with a new name shortly after this book is published.)

Page 5 *affecting more than 4.5 million children*
See, most recently: the Centers for Disease Control and Prevention statistics bulletin, at http://www.cdc.gov/ncbddd/adhd/data.html; as well as the August 2007 CDC e-newsletter, "Monitoring the Nation's Health," at www.cdc.gov.

Page 5 *including nearly one in ten boys*
The Centers for Disease Control and Prevention, in the report mentioned above, cites a diagnosis rate of nearly 8 percent, translating to

roughly 11 percent of U.S. boys, since boys are so much more commonly diagnosed than girls.

Page 5 *Japan and New Zealand*
See: Stephen V. Faraone, et al., "The Worldwide Prevalence of ADHD: Is It an American Condition?" *World Psychiatry* 2, no. 2 (June 2003): 104–113.

Page 5 *"dragon's bones"*
This bit of information comes from an interview with Dr. Yi Zheng, president of the Chinese Society for Child and Adolescent Psychiatry, courtesy of the Beijing-based independent journalist Kathleen McLaughlin.

Page 7 *four times as many car accidents . . . three times as likely to abuse alcohol and drugs*
These statistics come from a thoroughly harrowing lecture by the ADD expert Dr. Russell Barkley, which I attended at the University of California at Davis, on February 13, 2008.

Page 7 *$30 billion in above-the-norm annual medical expenses*
See: Howard G. Birnbaum et al., "Costs of Attention Deficit-Hyperactivity Disorder (ADHD) in the US: Excess Costs of Persons with ADHD and Their Family Members in 2000," *Current Medical Research and Opinion* 21, no. 2 (March 30, 2005): 195–205.

Page 8 *the provocateur and the easily provoked*
As Dr. Russell Barkley so eloquently writes in *Taking Charge of ADHD: The Complete, Authoritative Guide for Parents* (Guilford Press, 2000), the particular stress of having a child with ADD "is as great as or greater than that experienced by parents who have children with autism, a far more serious developmental disorder," in view of the "excessive, demanding, intrusive and generally high-intensity behavior . . . as well as their clear impairment in self-control."

1. HISTORY

Page 19 *In ancient Greece, impulsive behavior*
The Greek physician Hippocrates has been cited as having described a
condition similar to attention deficit disorder some 2,500 years ago.
See, for instance: A. Baumgaertel, "Alternative Controversial Treatments for Attention-Deficit/Hyperactivity Disorder," *Pediatric Clinics
of North America* 46, no. 5: 977–992, which says Hippocrates noted:
"quickened responses to sensory experience, but also less tenacious-
ness because the soul moves on quickly to the next impression,"
which he attributed to an "overbalance of fire over water."

Page 20 *Fidgety Phil*
"The Story of Fidgety Philip" is reprinted in Edward Hallowell and
John Ratey's *Driven to Distraction*:

> *"Let me see if Philip can*
> *Be a little gentleman;*
> *Let me see if he is able*
> *To sit still for once at the table."*
> *Thus Papa bade Phil behave;*
> *And Mama looked very grave.*
> *But Fidgety Phil,*
> *He won't sit still;*
> *He wriggles,*
> *And giggles,*
> *And then, I declare,*
> *Swings backwards and forwards,*
> *And tilts up his chair,*
> *Just like any rocking horse—*
> *"Philip! I am getting cross!"*
> *See the naughty, restless child*
> *Growing still more rude and wild,*
> *Till his chair falls over quite.*
> *Philip screams with all his might,*

Catches at the cloth, but then
That makes matters worse again.
Down upon the ground they fall,
Glasses, plates, knives, forks and all.
How Mama did fret and frown,
When she saw them tumbling down!
And Papa made such a face!
Philip is in sad disgrace . . .

Page 21 *and, naturally, lost it all*
My great-grandfather's spree is memorialized in *The Nine Lives of Michael Todd*, a biography of his celebrity nephew, by Art Cohn (Pocket Books, 1959).

Page 22 *killed as many as 40 million people*
See, for instance: http://virus.stanford.edu/uda/.

Page 22 *researchers dubbed this syndrome "postencephalitic behavior disorder"*
Much of this history is elaborated in Dr. Russell Barkley's *Taking Charge of ADHD*.

Page 24 *depression, drug abuse, or an eating disorder*
See, for instance: Joseph Biederman et al., "Are Girls with ADHD at Risk for Eating Disorders? Results from a Controlled, Five-Year Prospective Study," *Journal of Developmental & Behavioral Pediatrics* 28 (2007): 302. The authors reported that in a large study of adolescent girls with and without an attention disorder, those with the condition were nearly four times more likely to develop an eating disorder, defined as either anorexia or bulimia nervosa. Dr. Biederman's research has also shown that girls with ADD are more than five times more likely to develop major depression than girls without the disorder.

Page 26 *When she gave one boy a hug, he slapped her on her butt*
See: Maria Cook, "Young & Disorderly," *Ottawa Citizen*, December 9,

2001. This long profile includes some wonderful scenes from Douglas's research, including a description of how her team had to remove all the wheeled chairs from their lab, since the kids kept riding around on them, smashing into the computers.

Page 26 *"You wished you could get away with a lot of what they did"*

Douglas's seminal contribution to the field was her 1971 paper, entitled "Stop, Look and Listen: The Problem of Sustained Attention and Impulse Control in Hyperactive and Normal Children," *Canadian Journal of Behavioral Science* 4 (1972): 259–282. I interviewed her by telephone in the spring of 2008, when as an octogenarian she was still working in her clinic and writing research papers as an emeritus professor. In our conversation, she took pains to note her great admiration for her subjects' parents, who especially back in the 1970s and '80s had little idea what they were up against while in so many cases also struggling with similar issues as their children. "Some of them *drove* me places," she told me, with an audible shiver.

In the same interview Douglas also told me that she has felt somewhat responsible for, as well as conflicted about, the burgeoning trend of medicating children diagnosed with ADD, adding that she devoted much of her subsequent career to exploring alternatives, continually experimenting with behaviorally oriented programs emphasizing the practice of good habits and consistent rewards. "I wanted very, very badly to find ways other than stimulant medication to change these children," she said. "But nothing worked nearly as well."

Page 26 *prompted the $11 million lawsuit*

There's a long story here—so long that I once wrote an entire (and to date unpublished) book about it. To summarize, I was reporting on a murder-for-hire case in which the defendant, a man named Robert Singer, was charged with paying two young men to murder his wife's ex-husband. In a story on the final arguments, I incorrectly quoted a prosecutor as implicating Singer's wife, Judith Barnett, in the crime even though she had not been charged. I'm still not sure why I made this mistake, although some unconscious sense of justice may have been involved. At the time, it was an open secret that Barnett was having an affair with Singer's attorney, and many courtroom observers assumed she'd been the motivating force behind the plot to kill her ex-husband. The affair finally came to light—again, a long story, the highlight of which was that the defense attorney's secretary (who was angry at him, she said, for calling her "Fatso") sent me and Robert Singer a photocopied packet of explicit love letters, eventually prompting a retrial on the grounds of the attorney's clear conflict of interest. The revelations made Singer so angry that he testified against his wife, and in 1991, nearly a decade after the libel suit was filed and quickly dropped, Barnett was arrested and convicted in the murder. So there.

Page 28 *The series won a Pulitzer Prize*
Pete Carey, Lewis Simons, and I shared the award for the series, which was expertly guided by our editor, Jonathan Krim.

Page 30 *The drugs "make good caged animals"*
Dr. Breggin made this comment in a 2001 PBS *Frontline* report on "Medicating Kids." See: http://www.pbs.org/wgbh/pages/frontline/shows/medicating/interviews/breggin.html.

Page 30 *"end up abusing drugs"*
Many doctors have given this warning to mothers throughout the years, even as exhaustive research suggests it is unfounded. The largest study to date of this question found a neutral effect for medication in regards to later substance abuse. See: the editorial "Does Childhood Treatment of ADHD with Stimulant Medication Affect Substance Abuse in Adulthood?" *American Journal of Psychiatry* 165 (May 2008): 553–555.

Page 32 *babysitters quit on us*
Apparently, this is a global phenomenon. "Without Boundaries," an international survey of parents of ADD children directed by Dr. Russell

Barkley, showed that 46 percent of respondents reported they had troubles getting a babysitter, while 43 percent found it difficult to appear in public with their child, and 32 percent felt uncomfortable inviting friends and family to their home because of the child's symptoms. Meanwhile, about half of the parents believed their marriage had been negatively affected, rising to about two-thirds in the United Kingdom and Australia. The report can be found at www.ldaa.ca/assets/pdfs/freeresources/ADHDWithout Boundaries.pdf.

Page 33 *"Open to experience . . ."*
Jim's joke arose from a typically ADD cognitive detour. My impending operation had inspired a conversation with him about "trepanning," an ancient practice in which a hole is cut into the skull in pursuit of medical or spiritual benefits. There've even been a few modern proponents of trepanning, including the Dutch librarian and former medical student Bart Huges, who theorized that children whose skulls are not fully closed have a higher state of consciousness. Huges championed trepanation in his 1962 monograph *Homo Sapiens Correctus.*

2. EMERGENCY

Page 36 *frying latkes with my friend Sally*
I've changed my friends' names and professions, but all the other details are true.

Page 38 *a reported 2.5 million U.S. children*
This estimate is from the Centers for Disease Control and Prevention. See, for example: "Mental Health in the United States: Prevalence of Diagnosis and Medication Treatment for Attention-Deficit/ Hyperactivity Disorder—United States, 2003," *MMWR Weekly* 54, no. 34 (September 2, 2005): 842–847.

Page 38 *a Rhode Island institute*

This was the Emma Pendleton Bradley Institute, established through the will of George Bradley, a wealthy businessman whose daughter had suffered from epilepsy and mental retardation.

Page 38 *a specially designed chair*

Dr. Glen Elliott of the Children's Health Council in Palo Alto, California, kindly provided this description of the pneumoencephalogram.

Page 38 *the medication instead improved their focus and self-control*

U.S. researchers of the 1950s were unconstrained by today's ethical standards, which strictly limit experiments on humans. In that absence, researchers at the Bradley home were free to run tests on their wards that would never be possible today, for good reason, even as they increased understanding of the mechanics of ADD. In one, described by Dr. Russell Barkley in *Attention-Deficit Hyperactivity Disorder: A Handbook for Diagnosis and Treatment* (Guilford Press, 2006), Maurice Laufer, then staff director of the Bradley Institute, and colleagues, gave children varying doses of a drug called metronidazole, used today mainly to treat bacterial infections and parasites, and which has side effects including headaches, loss of appetite, and, more rarely, seizures and nerve damage. They then hooked up their subjects to EEG machines and flashed a light in their eyes, inducing their muscles to jerk in reflex. Laufer reported that children with hyperactivity required less of the drug to elicit the jerk than those without, suggesting a lower threshold for stimulation. Laufer's new paradigm helped move future researchers toward a model of a disorder based on brain dynamics, which helped lead to a 1968 decision by the American Psychiatric Association (APA) to rename the disorder that eventually became known as ADD as "hyperkinetic reaction of childhood."

Page 39 *nearly tripled in size worldwide between 1993 and 2007*

See: Yasmin Anwar, "Use of ADHD Medication Soars World-

wide," *U.C. Berkeley News,* March 6, 2007, http://berkeley.edu/news/
media/releases/2007/03/06_adhd.shtml.

Page 39 *Americans spent $291 billion on prescription drugs
in 2008*
This estimate comes from the IMS Health market research firm and
is available in a report at http://www.imshealth.com/portal/site/im
shealth/menuitem.a46c6d4df3db4b3d88f611019418c22a/?vgnextoid=
85f4a56216a10210VgnVCM100000ed152ca2RCRD&cpsextcur
rchannel=1.

Page 39 *nearly 65 percent of us, and increasingly also our cats
and dogs*
See: Melody Petersen, *Our Daily Meds: How the Pharmaceutical
Companies Transformed Themselves into Slick Marketing Machines
and Hooked the Nation on Prescription Drugs* (Farrar, Straus and
Giroux 2008).

Page 39 *U.S. children are three times more likely to be treated
with stimulants*
Julie M. Zito et al., "A Three-Country Comparison of Psychotropic
Medication Prevalence in Youth," *Child and Adolescent Psychiatry
and Mental Health* 2 (September 2008): 26. Also worth noting is
that in the United Kingdom, official health guidelines issued in
September 2008 recommended that children be treated with medications only in severe cases and never when they are younger than
five.

Pages 39–40 *Medication proved better than behavior therapy*
See: http://www.ncbi.nlm.nih.gov/pubmed/11265923. The MTA study
involved nearly six hundred children assigned to groups receiving
four different types of treatments: behavior therapy, rigorously supervised medication, a combination of both, and "community care"—
i.e., the prevailing U.S. standard of care, which most often amounts to
lightly supervised medication. Its conclusion: the combination of meds

and behavioral therapy works best, but if you can't do both, choose the meds.

(William Pelham, a professor of psychology at the University at Buffalo, and one of the authors of the report, described himself to me as one of its few outspoken in-house critics. He keenly prefers behavioral therapy over drugs whenever possible, believing it to be both more effective and safer in the long run. Yet even Pelham acknowledged that nothing beats the meds in a crisis. "If I were kidnapped today by a Middle Eastern terrorist and taken to Abu Dhabi with a gun to my head and ordered to make my kidnapper's son normal right away, I'd ask if he had any Concerta," he quipped.)

Page 40 *nearly 60 percent of U.S. kids diagnosed with attention deficit disorder*
Visser, Lesesne, and Perou, "National Estimates and Factors Associated with Medication Treatment for Childhood Attention-Deficit/Hyperactivity Disorder," *Pediatrics* 119 (2007): 99–106.

Page 40 *earning less than the so-called living wage*
Barbara Ehrenreich, *Nickel and Dimed: On (Not) Getting By in America* (Metropolitan Books, 2001).

Page 40 *Dr. Harold Koplewicz*
Dr. Lawrence Diller features this quote in his book *The Last Normal Child* (Greenwood Publishing Group, 2006). I interviewed Dr. Koplewicz myself on January 21, 2009. During our conversation, he initially agreed that the quote was correct, but then said he may have been taken out of context and was speaking to the case of parents who refuse to offer *any* treatment for their children with ADHD. He offered to establish this by sending me his tape of the interview, but I didn't hear from him again after that. By the way, Dr. Koplewicz was on the board of Eli Lilly when he made his comment in the ABC-TV interview. He said he later quit, after accepting what he estimates was no more than $22,000 from drug firms during his

career, adding that he ceased any involvement with them as of circa 2002, so as to be more credible with the public.

Page 40 *the Ritalin Wars*
Critics of the widespread use of Ritalin have rightly pointed out that the rates of diagnoses and treatment throughout America vary unsettlingly from place to place. (The American Academy of Pediatrics has found a range of from 4 to 12 percent of children being diagnosed, depending on the location.) To me, this suggests that some children are probably being medicated unnecessarily, even as others may not be getting the help they need.

Page 41 *not a single close friend*
In his lecture at the University of California at Davis, Dr. Russell Barkley said that a child with ADD is "likely to be friendless" by second or third grade.

Page 42 *more than twice as likely to separate or divorce*
See, for example: "Couples with Children with ADHD at Risk of Higher Divorce Rates, Shorter Marriages," *Medical News Today,* October 22, 2008. Dr. Russell Barkley gives a higher estimate of divorce rates in his *Taking Charge of ADHD* (Guilford Press, 2000).

Page 43 *including Novartis, Shire, McNeil Pediatrics, and Eli Lilly*
The disclosure of financial interests in these and other companies by researchers involved in the 1999 study was sixty-one lines long.

Page 43 *paid adviser to six drug companies, a paid speaker for six companies, and a paid researcher for ten companies*
This comes from Dr. Biederman's disclosure in an article he authored for *Medscape,* published July 18, 2006: "The Effects of Attention-Deficit/Hyperactivity Disorder on Employment and Household Income." Dr. Biederman's ties with drug firms were also featured in a *New York Times* article on June 8, 2008: "Researchers Fail to Reveal

Full Drug Pay," by Gardiner Harris and Benedict Carey. The report revealed that U.S. congressional investigators had charged Dr. Biederman with failing to disclose $1.6 million in drug money.

When I interviewed Dr. Biederman in July of 2008, he called the investigation "a public lynching." Drug companies and the researchers they pay deserve more gratitude than distrust, he insisted. "It costs a billion dollars to get a medication to market, and there is no other way to do that without a drug company," Dr. Biederman told me. "And there is simply no question that medications have improved our lives, and saved lives. Longevity has increased by twenty years in modern times, and I can assure you that's not because of the weather." When it came to ADD, he said, his critics weren't considering the substantial risks of bad outcomes, including "school failure, drug abuse, nicotine abuse, you name it," when they "demonized" drugs that he insisted were as safe as asthma inhalers.

Page 43 *nearly a quarter of his 2007 income from ADD drug manufacturers*
Dr. Barkley disclosed his income sources on his Web site, http://www.russellbarkley.org/, which I accessed in June 2009.

Page 43 *Dr. Edward Hallowell, who touted methylphenidate*
See: the McNeil press release of September 18, 2008, "National Survey Reveals Impact of ADHD in Adults," http://www.add.org/pdf/Adult_ADHD_Survey.pdf.

Page 44 *refuted by U.S. federal investigators*
The Texas study raised suspicions early on—see Gardiner Harris, "Report of Ritalin Prompts a Federal Study," *New York Times,* July 1, 2005—but the final government determination that refuted it was never prominently reported. In 2008, I interviewed Dr. David Jacobson-Kram of the Office of New Drugs at the FDA, who had investigated the conclusions. He told me there were serious issues with the way the study had been conducted, and that a larger German review had credibly dismissed its conclusions.

Page 44 *stimulants stunt growth*

See, for instance: "Treatment of ADHD: Some Good News, Some Bad," *Neuropsychiatry Review* 5, no. 4 (June 2004).

Page 44 *mixed bag of anti-drug crusaders*

Consider, for instance, the Web site www.ritalindeath.com, which makes the baseless charge that "thousands of children have died over the years as a direct result of using psychotropic drugs for ADD," and the energetic Beaverton, Oregon, vitamin and e-book salesman Jon Bennett, who in 2008 claimed 147,000 subscribers to his Web site, touting "3 Steps to Conquering ADD-ADHD." (In e-mails declaring, "This is what the Big Drug companies don't want you to know!" Bennett has acknowledged he has no medical background—"If you want some hoity-toity Doctor guru guy, you are going to be disappointed." He bases his expertise instead on the fact that he "grew up in an ADD ADHD home" and watched his brother Jeremy take medication, after which, "overnight I saw his personality totally change from a fun-loving kid into a zombie.")

Page 44 *significantly more likely than peers to be physically harmed by their frustrated parents*

In June 2008, I spoke with Michael Haney, director of child abuse programs for the Florida Department of Health, who said a majority of parental abuse cases he saw involved children with ADD. "They're extremely challenging children, and if you combine poor parenting skills, it's a dangerous match," Haney said, adding that such incidents were on the increase as the U.S. economy worsened.

I was able to find just one study on this topic, however, by ADD researcher Stephen Hinshaw and colleagues, in the journal *Child Abuse and Neglect* 30, no. 11 (November 2006): 1239–1255. The researchers found significantly higher rates of physical abuse for girls with ADD, at 14.3 percent, compared with a control group of girls, at 4.5 percent, but, significantly, did not determine whether the abuse was triggered by the ADD or whether ADD may have aggravated it.

Page 44 *shipping their unmanageable offspring off*
Lower-income parents have fewer options but can be just as desperate, as was revealed in 2008, during my year of paying attention to attention, when thirty-five children were dropped off by their guardians with state officials in Nebraska, taking advantage of a temporary loophole in a law meant to protect unwanted infants.

Page 46 *"like Benny Schwartz gets"*
Benny Schwartz is a pseudonym.

Page 47 *Peter Breggin*
While deepening my research into ADD and Ritalin, I'd learned more about Dr. Breggin, who never responded to my several requests for an interview. I'd read how he'd first become justifiably distressed over the treatment of psychiatric patients as a teaching fellow at Harvard Medical School in the 1960s, back in that *One Flew Over the Cuckoo's Nest* era of locked wards and electroshock treatments, yet how his ire at conventional psychiatry later led him to unstinting and, according to his critics, reckless opposition of the large and growing body of research establishing the predominantly biochemical nature of mental illness. For a time, Dr. Breggin was allied with the Church of Scientology, a group that he and his wife Ginger eventually renounced.

Dr. Breggin's erstwhile colleagues have condemned him for seeming to suggest even severely mentally disordered patients shouldn't be taking medication. Leaders of U.S. psychiatric associations have called him "ignorant" and an "outlaw." Judges have rebuked him in at least three legal actions, accusing him of being "unqualified," a "fraud," and compromised by "blinding" bias. (See: Christine Gorman et al., "Prozac's Worst Enemy," *Time*, Monday, October 10, 1994).

Page 48 *Tyrannosaurus rex*
Ilina Singh, "Bad Boys, Good Mothers, and the 'Miracle' of Ritalin," *Science in Context* 15 (2002): 577–603.

Page 50 *even improvement in the mothers' relationships with their husbands, and their sons' teachers*

Singh, "Doing Their Jobs: Mothering with Ritalin in a Culture of Mother-Blame," *Social Science & Medicine* 59 (2004): 1193–1205.

See also: A. Chronis-Tuscano et al., "Efficacy of Osmotic-Release Oral System (OROS) Methylphenidate for Mothers with Attention Deficity/Hyperactivity Disorder," *Journal of Clinical Psychiatry* 69, no. 12 (December 2008): 1938–1947. The lead author, Dr. Chronis-Tuscano, did not respond to several calls and e-mails, but Concerta spokeswoman Trish Geoghegan told me that McNeil Pediatrics, the manufacturer of Concerta, paid for this study.

Page 50 *About 85 percent have a positive reaction*

These statistics come from an interview in February 2008 with Dr. Glen Elliott at the Children's Health Council in Palo Alto, California. See also: "Rationale, Design, and Methods of the Preschool ADHD Treatment Study," *Journal of the American Academy of Child & Adolescent Psychiatry* 45, no. 11 (November 2006): 1275–1283.

Page 50 *various side effects*

Marcia L. Buck, "Methylphenidate: New Information and New Options," *Pediatric Pharmacotherapy* 8, no. 2 (2002).

---

3. BIOLOGY

Page 55 *"Biobabble"*

This is a quote from the British psychiatrist Sami Timimi (www .psychminded.co.uk).

Page 55 *"The disease du jour"* . . . *"A neat way to explain the complexities of turn-of-the-millennium life in America"*

These quotes are from the educator and psychologist Thomas Armstrong, whose Web site is http://www.thomasarmstrong.com/myth_ add_adhd.htm.

Page 55 *no blood test or even brain scan*

In the year 2000, Xavier Castellanos, then head of ADD research at the National Institute of Mental Health, acknowledged in an interview with PBS TV ("Medicating Young Minds") that there was no "objective way" of diagnosing the disorder, "because we don't really understand what it is." As I've researched this book, other equally candid experts have agreed that not much had changed since then.

Page 55 *a checklist of behaviors*

Many children and adults being diagnosed today, by family doctors and pediatricians, are told they have attention deficit disorder, or attention deficit/hyperactivity disorder. A more thorough evaluation, from a psychiatrist or psychologist, however, might lead to a classification under one of three "subtypes" of the disorder, as elaborated in the fourth edition of the *Diagnostic and Statistical Manual of Mental Disorders*. The subtypes are attention-deficit/hyperactivity disorder, combined type; attention-deficit/hyperactivity disorder, predominantly inattentive type; and attention-deficit/hyperactivity disorder, predominantly hyperactive-impulsive type.

For the inattentive subtype, six or more of the following symptoms must have been present for at least six months to a "maladaptive" degree:

1. Often fails to give close attention to details or makes careless mistakes in schoolwork, work, or other activities.
2. Often has trouble keeping attention in tasks or play activities.
3. Often does not seem to listen when spoken to directly.
4. Often does not follow through on instructions and fails to finish schoolwork, chores, or duties in the workplace (not due to oppositional behavior or failure to understand instructions).
5. Often has difficulty organizing tasks and activities.
6. Often avoids, dislikes, or is reluctant to engage in tasks that require sustained mental effort (such as schoolwork or homework).

7. Often loses things needed for tasks and activities (e.g., toys, school assignments, pencils, books, or tools).

8. Is often easily distracted by extraneous stimuli.

9. Is often forgetful in daily activities.

For the hyperactive-impulsive type, the key symptoms are:

1. Often fidgets with hands or feet or squirms in seat.

2. Often leaves seat in classroom or in other situations in which remaining seated is expected.

3. Often runs about or climbs excessively in situations in which it is inappropriate (in adolescents or adults, may be limited to subjective feelings of restlessness).

4. Often has difficulty playing or enjoying leisure activities quietly.

5. Is often "on the go" or often acts as if "driven by a motor."

6. Often talks excessively.

Specific symptoms of impulsivity are:

1. Often blurts out answers before questions have been finished.

2. Often has difficulty awaiting turn.

3. Often interrupts or intrudes on others (e.g., butts into conversations or games).

Page 56 *Several brain structures are on average as much as 12 percent smaller . . .*

I relied on several sources for this overview, including telephone interviews with Dr. Russell Barkley and, at the National Institutes of Mental Health, Dr. Philip Shaw, and these written materials: Joel T. Nigg, *What Causes ADHD?* (Guilford Press, 2006), pp. 54–61; Valera et al., "Meta-analysis of Structural Imaging Findings in Attention-Deficit/ Hyperactivity Disorder," *Biological Psychiatry* 61, no. 12 (June 15, 2007): 1361–1369; "Brain Shrinkage in ADHD not Caused by Medications," National Institutes of Health news release, October 8, 2002; Katya Rubia et al., "Neuroanatomic Evidence for the Maturational Delay Hypothesis of Attention Deficit Hyperactivity Disorder,"

Proceedings of the National Academy of Sciences 104, no. 50 (December 11, 2007), 19663–19664; and "Brain Matures a Few Years Late in ADHD, but Follows Normal Pattern," *NIH News,* November 12, 2007.

Page 56 *frontal lobes*

To illustrate how the state of the frontal lobes can determine someone's personality, neuroscientists love to tell the story of Phineas Gage, a railroad worker who in the summer of 1871 was most definitely in the wrong place at the wrong time. In the midst of a badly organized effort to blast through rock in the way of a new track in Vermont, a long steel "tamping rod" used to compress a charge of gunpowder was sent flying straight through Gage's skull. He miraculously survived, but his personality was transformed. As his doctor, John Harlow, later famously recalled, Gage, by all accounts previously amiable and hardworking, lost the "balance . . . between his intellectual faculty and animal propensities," leaving him "fitful, irreverent, indulging at times in the grossest profanity (which was not previously his custom), manifesting little deference to his fellows, impatient of restraint or advice when it conflicts with his desires, at times pertinaciously obstinate, yet capricious and vacillating, devising many plans of future operation, which are no sooner arranged than they are abandoned."

Gage's altered temperament led to his ruin. He was fired, shunned, and according to Harlow, ended up parading his injury at P. T. Barnum's New York museum and working at odd jobs for the next twelve years before his death.

Page 56 *"sleepy" brains*

I first heard the more precise term, "sleepy cortex," from Dr. John Ratey, a Cambridge psychiatrist and coauthor of *Driven to Distraction* (Touchstone, 1994).

Page 56 *ADD brains* crave *it*

Dr. Daniel Amen observantly notes that people with ADD like to play a game called "Let's Have a Problem." He told me that many mothers of his patients say their kids have some of their best days at school after revving up their brains with nagging and fights in the morning.

Page 57 *ADD brains have a major problem with this vital chemical*

In September 2009, an eight-year study led to a breakthrough report on this line of research: Nora D. Volkow, M.D., et al., "Evaluating Dopamine Reward Pathway in ADHD," *Journal of the American Medical Association* 302, no. 10 (2009): 1084–1091. I reported on the JAMA study for the *Washington Post*, in a story headlined "Brain Scans Link ADHD to Biological Flaw Tied to Motivation," September 22, 2009.

Page 57 *a family legacy*

My brief description of ADD gene research owes mostly to the generosity of Susan Smalley, PhD, a professor in the Department of Psychiatry and Biobehavioral Sciences at the University of California at Los Angeles, whom I interviewed in February 2008. Smalley specializes in the genetics of psychiatric disorders, with a special emphasis on ADD. Her research team is focused on searching among the approximately 25,000 genes in the human genome for those that may contribute to clinical distraction. Recent advances in molecular genetics have facilitated this search, in particular by detecting something called SNPS, single nucleotide polymorphisms, which are variations in DNA sequences that occur periodically along the human genome. SNPS are markers for diseases and disorders. Sometimes they contribute to causing those problems; other times they merely point the way to the gene variations that do, and thus help narrow down what would otherwise have been an overwhelming search.

Smalley's investigators collect samples of blood and saliva from volunteers from families with ADD symptoms—preferably from siblings with many genes in common. They can then find SNPS in

common, leading them to the genes that may be involved in the distraction.

Page 57 *helped our primitive hunter ancestors survive*
Thom Hartman, *Beyond ADD: Hunting for Reasons in the Past and
Present* (Underwood Books, 1996).

Page 58 *descendants of the tribes that crossed over the Bering
Straits*
For a more thorough explanation of this fascinating detour, see: Peter
C. Whybrow, *American Mania: When More Is Not Enough* (W.W.
Norton & Company, 2005).

Page 60 *as I sat cowering on my aluminum chair*
Dr. Barkley has collected his statistics since 1978, in the Milwaukee
Longitudinal Study. His research includes periodic observations of
239 children, 158 of whom have been diagnosed with ADD, as they
grow to adulthood. His work is extraordinary, solid, and compelling,
which of course makes it all the more depressing.

Page 61 *"archaic, dated, and stupid"*
This quote is from an excellent profile of Dr. Amen by Mary Sykes
Wylie, entitled "Visionary or Voodoo?" in *Psychotherapy Networker,*
September/October 2005.

Page 61 *"led by God"*
Ibid.

Page 62 *a paper denouncing the use of SPECT*
Dr. Amen responded to the rebuke with a letter, signed by thirty-six
other MDs and PhDs, calling the report biased and wrong. In particular, he said, it wasn't right to imply that he used his scans to make
diagnoses. Rather, he said, the best use of those images is "to add
functional data" to his clinical work.

(Judging from my own experience, however, this does seem a bit like splitting hairs. Functional data or diagnoses—what does it matter if the scans aren't valid? And when he told me, "There's your ADD!" wasn't that a diagnosis?)

Page 63 *"no evidence that would suggest that these substances would work as a brain supplement"*
"Really? Not even the GABA?" I asked McGaugh at the time. It seemed so plausible that GABA, or gamma-aminobutryic acid, an important neurotransmitter, might help, since, rather than influencing forward motion, like dopamine, GABA involves inhibition—those mental brakes. But McGaugh burst my bubble. "We've obtained quite a bit of evidence that drugs that promote GABA impair memory," he told me. "So you may feel better on it, with less anxiety, but you'll be storing less information while under the drug, so there's a price to pay." In other words, the GABA might initially make me less anxious, but messing with my already problematic memory would likely guarantee more anxiety down the line.

Page 73 *as if it's all coming easily to him*
The educational counselor Meredith Warshaw has an extremely helpful site compiling advice for parents of "twice-exceptional children," at http://www.uniquelygifted.org/.

Page 73 *Working memory*
Just for fun, my brother Jim e-mailed me his own favorite example of a working-memory test, from an old Danny Kaye movie, *The Court Jester,* in which Kaye plays a character on a life-or-death mission, the outcome of which depends on his keeping in mind a complicated series of instructions. It begins: "The pellet with the poison's in the vessel with the pestle; the chalice from the palace has the brew that is true—" yet must be constantly adjusted, as for instance, the chalice is broken and must be replaced with "a flagon, with the figure of a dragon. . . ."

Page 75 *except for looking into further meds, at least for now*
This wasn't as quick a decision as it may seem. In fact, I spent considerable time over the subsequent two weeks pestering Brown for more details about the source of her concern about Buzz's emotional state—until she finally conceded that she was relying mostly on *Rorschach blots*. That's right, those ink splotches you see the mad psychiatrists waving around in black-and-white movies from the 1940s. This turn-of-the-century diagnostic tool, the brainchild of the Swiss Freudian psychiatrist Hermann Rorschach, is as controversial as it stubbornly remains iconic, in our dawning molecular-based view of the brain. I mean, just think about it. A patient interprets an image. The therapist interprets the interpretation. What could be more subjective? My confidence in Brown somewhat shaken, I switched to full-scale reporter mode and kept bugging her until she agreed to check her notes for the interpretations Buzz made that so worried her. It turned out he'd described one blot as "a pissed-off bird," and another as "a sad, flowered face." Downbeat as these observations seemed, they didn't persuade me that more meds were required.

Page 76 *"penis deficit/hypermammary disorder"*
See: "An Interview with Laura Honos-Webb," at http://www.new harbinger.com/client/client_pages/honoswebbtinterview.cfm.

---

4. RELATIONSHIPS

Page 77 *documented adolescent diurnal rhythms*
See, for instance: Claudia Wallis, "What Makes Teens Tick," *Time*, May 10, 2004.

Page 81 *an equally murky prism*
For an interesting take on ODD, see Marc Bousquet, "Oppositional and Defiant—Or Critical Thinker?" *Chronicle of Higher Education*,

September 12, 2008. (Bousquet quotes one wry commentator as writing, "Finally, a cure for the class struggle.")

Page 82 *The Nurture Assumption*
Some prominent U.S. psychologists have accused Harris of ignoring studies that didn't support her thesis, and misinterpreting important evidence.

Page 82 *Michael Meany's pioneering discovery*
Ethan Watters, "DNA Is Not Destiny," *Discover*, November 22, 2006.

Jim Robbins, in *A Symphony in the Brain: The Evolution of the New Brain Wave Biofeedback* (Grove Press, 2008), describes how a similar phenomenon appears to affect humans, according to a University of Minnesota study that showed that children who have a poor emotional attachment to their parents get higher rushes of cortisol during even mildly painful events, such as being vaccinated, than do children with strong parental bonds.

Page 82 *Michael Posner*
See: Posner's Seventy-seventh James Arthur Lecture "On the Evolution of the Human Brain," March 20, 2007.

Also of interst is: L.A. Tully et al., "Does Maternal Warmth Moderate the Effects of Birth Weight on Twins' Attention-Deficit/ Hyperactivity Disorder (ADHD) Symptoms and Low IQ?" *Journal of Consulting and Clinical Psychology* 72, no. 2 (April 2004): 218–226. This research has shown that more engaged and affectionate mothers can actually reduce the degree of ADD symptoms in low-birth-weight babies, who are at greater risk for the disorder. And herein lies a tale.

Terrie Moffitt, now at Duke University, released this finding in 2004, based on a study of 2,232 five-year-old twins, half of whom had low birth weight. In an interview in 2008, she told me that her report sparked a backlash that surprised her. The immediate criticism included a letter from Dr. Russell Barkley, who accused Moffitt of "investigator bias" and of unfairly blaming mothers. Moffitt and her colleagues defended the research at the time but never followed up on it. "We just thought, why continue to fight this?" Moffitt told me.

Page 83 *the "normal" mothers were pestering*
From Hugh Lytton, "Child and Parent Effects in Boys' Conduct Disorder: A Reinterpretation," *Developmental Psychology* 26, no. 5 (1990): 683–697.

Page 83 *The child's extraordinary resistance*
For research on this, see, for example: J. D. Burke et al., "Reciprocal Relationships Between Parenting Behavior and Disruptive Psychopathology from Childhood Through Adolescence," *Journal of Abnormal Child Psychology* 36, no. 5 (July 2008): 679–692. The authors said they found "greater influence of child behaviors on parenting behaviors than of parenting behaviors on child behaviors." In particular, they said, "unpleasant child behaviors coerce parents to discontinue engaging in appropriate discipline," in which case "timid discipline predicted worsening behavior, namely ODD symptoms, and ODD symptoms predicted (further) increases in timid discipline."

Page 83 *until everything falls apart*
The danger is particularly acute in families in which both parents and children are clinically distracted. See, for example: "Relationship of Family Environment and Parental Psychiatric Diagnosis to Impairment in ADHD," *Journal of the American Academy of Child and Adolescent Psychiatry,* March 2006. The authors found that children who grow up with clinically distracted parents are more likely to suffer higher rates of family conflict and lower rates of cohesion, or capacity to stick by one another, leaving children more likely to be anxious, addicted, and abusive.

Page 84 *"a caricature of a bad fifth-grade schoolteacher"*
See: Edward Hallowell and John Ratey, *Delivered from Distraction:*

Getting the Most Out of Life with Attention Deficit Disorder (Ballantine Books, 2005).

Page 86 *bruises, cuts, chipped teeth, and broken bones*
Katy Butler, "Beyond Rivalry, a Hidden World of Sibling Violence," *New York Times*, February 28, 2006.

Page 94 *Benny Bolansky*
A pseudonym.

---

5. SOCIETY

Page 99 *a form of that stillness*
The quote is from Josef Pieper's *Leisure: The Basis of Culture* (1952), cited by David Levy in his essay "No Time to Think." (The essay is published in the online journal *Ethics and Information Technology*, http://www.springerlink.com/content/q5154248132321tn/.) Levy is a leader of the rebel forces against overbusyness. As founder of the Center for Information and the Quality of Life at the University of Washington, he's linked in with the increasing global campaigns to "unplug," buy fewer things, eat more slowly, take vacations, and celebrate Sabbaths, secular and sacred. He compares the emerging backlash to the birth of the environmental movement—a similar critique of capitalism, with its idea that ever more consumption, in this case including consumption of data, automatically increases well-being.

Page 101 *"An explosive outburst"*
See: Ross Greene's landmark book, *The Explosive Child*, first published in 1998.

Page 102 *falling into the same hole*
This is a reference to Portia Nelson's "Autobiography in Five Short Chapters," which I found in its entirety at http://www.lessons4 living.com/sidewalk_of_life.htm.

Page 104 *a constant flow of external temptations*
Just consider: by 2003, 55 percent of U.S. homes were connected to
the Internet, with more than four in ten Americans using the Web at
work. ("Computer and Internet Use in the United States: 2003," U.S.
Census Bureau report, 2005.)

At last count, more than 70 million blogs and 150 million Web
sites were competing to tell us something we didn't yet know, with
the number of these pages expanding at the rate of ten thousand an
hour. By one recent estimate (see: Bree Nordenson, "Overload! Journalism's Battle for Relevance in an Age of Too Much Information,"
Columbia Journalism Review, November/December 2008), 210 billion e-mails are sent each day, carrying news of Nigerian financial
scams, reports of oppressed Burmese monks, and cathartic missives
from friends who, before e-mail, would surely have waited to talk in
person.

Page 104 *superior colliculus*
Paul G. Overton, "Collicular Dysfunction in Attention Deficit Hyperactivity Disorder," *Medical Hypotheses* 70 (2008): 1121–1127.

Page 105 *we multitask by toggling between endeavors*
This is according to the University of Michigan cognitive scientist
David Meyer, an international expert on multitasking whom I inter-
viewed in late 2008.

Page 105 *955 deaths and 240,000 accidents*
Matt Richtel, "U.S. Withheld Data on Risks of Distracted Driving,"
New York Times, July 20, 2009.

Page 105 *as they would if they smoked dope*
"'Infomania' Worse Than Marijuana," BBC News, April 22, 2005.

(In a Harris poll in 2004, nine out of ten respondents claimed
they multitasked, while nearly six in ten said they were getting less
done.)

Page 106 *a "frenetic chase"*

Quoted in Peter C. Whybrow, *American Mania: When More Is Not Enough* (W.W. Norton & Co., 2005).

Page 108 *the cognitive rewards, with flashing graphics and noise, are immediate and addictive*

See, for instance: David Derbyshire, "Social Websites Harm Children's Brains: Chilling Warning to Parents from Top Neuroscientist," *Mail Online,* February 24, 2009.

And also: Claudia Wallis, "The Multitasking Generation," *Time,* March 19, 2006, which describes how family interactions are eroding as parents and kids get increasingly absorbed in their gadgets.

Page 109 *the alarming "nature deficit"*

See: Richard Louv, *Last Child in the Woods: Saving Our Children from Nature-Deficit Disorder* (Atlantic Books, 2005).

Page 113 *I eventually do quit the parent-teacher council*

An additional human-nature problem that I would have elaborated on in the main text if the chapter hadn't been getting so darn long, is the strong drive to keep options open, even when it's clear we should be closing some doors. The *New York Times* columnist John Tierney wrote a wonderful column about this entitled "The Advantages of Closing a Few Doors," published on February 26, 2008, in which he described research led by Dan Ariely, a professor of Behavioral Economics at the Massachusetts Institute of Technology. Ariely conducted an experiment in which hundreds of students were taught to play a computer game in which they were paid real cash to look for virtual money behind three doors on a screen. To boil down the findings: students fiercely resisted abandoning doors that started to fade away, even as keeping them open was clearly against their economic interests. "Closing a door on an option is experienced as a loss, and people are willing to pay a price to avoid the emotion of loss," Dr. Ariely told Tierney.

Page 114 *Max is in the back next to Andy . . . and his brother Stephen*

Andy and Stephen are aliases.

Page 116 *"knots to undo"*

This is from the book *Bar Mitzvah: A Guide to Spiritual Growth,* by Marc-Alain Ouaknin and Francoise-Anne Menager (Assouline, 2005).

---

6. EDUCATION

Page 117 *a special summer school class on brain science*

The name of the program is BWH ScienceWorks.

Page 119 *constant risk of tuning out or acting up*

Studies show that a high-quality connection with a teacher is the most powerful spur for academic success—as well as for avoiding failures such as drug abuse, delinquency, and dropouts. See, for instance: Wigfield, et al., "The Development of Children's Motivation in School Contexts," *Review of Research in Education* 23, no. 1 (1998): 73–118. And also: Malcolm Gladwell, "Most Likely to Succeed," *New Yorker,* December 15, 2008. Gladwell quotes Stanford economist Eric Hanushek as saying that the United States could close the gap between higher-achieving education systems such as those in Canada and Belgium just by replacing the bottom 6 percent to 10 percent of public school teachers with teachers of average quality. Gladwell's article joins the chorus of advocates for dramatic rethinking in teacher hiring and promotions, as he argues that teachers should be judged and rewarded according to their success in the classroom.

Page 119 *famously bad for boys*

See, for instance: Peg Tyre, *The Trouble with Boys: A Surprising Report Card on Our Sons, Their Problems at School, and What Parents and Educators Must Do* (Crown, 2008). Tyre reports that although boys and girls have similar IQ levels, boys are disengaging from the educational process earlier on, and falling further behind each year. Boys, she writes, are being "expelled" from preschool at a rate four times that of girls, are 60 percent more likely to be held back in kindergarten, and are twice as likely to be diagnosed with a learning disability.

Page 119 *as many as 40 percent will drop out*
Dr. Russell Barkley confirmed this to me in an e-mail on October 28, 2009.

Page 121 *dopamine glitch*
See: Joel T. Nigg, *What Causes ADHD?* (Guilford Press, 2006).

Page 123 *the Bermuda Triangle of American education*
Claudia Wallis, "Is Middle School Bad for Kids?" *Time,* August 1, 2005.

Page 124 *waiting for something to happen*
See: Philip Jackson, *Life in Classrooms* (Teachers College Press, 1990).

Page 126 *in return for larger classes, lower test scores, and higher drop-out rates*
Paul Basken, "Asia Gains on U.S., Europe in Education, OECD Finds," Bloomberg, September 12, 2006.

Page 127 *"zero tolerance" for behaviors*
These more punitive policies amount to a de facto exclusion of students with problems such as ADD, who often end up in alternative placements that are academically inferior or more expensive, and sometimes both, according to psychology professor Steven Evans, at the James Madison University in Virginia, who has studied these issues extensively, and whom I interviewed in May of 2009.

Also see: "Zero Tolerance Policies and the Public Schools: When Suspension Is No Longer Effective," *NASP Communique* 37, no. 5 (January/February 2009). The article notes that even as schools commonly justify strict suspension and expulsion policies as needed to curb violence, nine out of ten of them report they have no serious violent crimes, while 99 percent of students overall don't commit serious crimes in school.

Page 127 *explaining how to use* "me gusta"
Every once in a while, on my middle school parent-teacher council, someone would ask what teachers were doing to encourage gifted students. The answer was always the same: the teachers had been trained in "differentiated learning," we were told, meaning that they knew how to adjust their teaching to their students' skill level. Anyone probing further, however, would find that what this meant was that kids who showed extra talent and finished their worksheets quickly would be handed "extra credit" worksheets. "That's like punishing them, isn't it?" one observant parent asked. Buzz seemed to agree; he never did the extra work.

My worry is that kids like Buzz, with quick comprehension but slow self-control, have become a dramatically underserved minority in U.S. schools, where the doctrine of "leave no child behind" devotes the lion's share of resources to children with garden-variety difficulties in understanding the curriculum, slow learners and non-native English speakers. In our current education crisis, the idea of "pushing some kids ahead" is seen as a luxury, despite all we know about how chronically bored kids are extra-vulnerable to problems such as drug abuse.

Page 127 *"if the schools were okay, we wouldn't need meds"*
Dr. Peter Breggin made the same point, in more aggressive terms, on the 2001 PBS program "Medicating Kids," saying the meds facilitate "the smooth functioning of overstressed families and schools. . . . It's about having submissive children who will sit in a

boring classroom of thirty, often with teachers who don't know how
to use visual aids and all the other exciting technologies that kids
are used to."

Page 129 *The first High Tech High school opened in 2000*
Grace Rubenstein, "Hands-on Learning at High Tech High,"
Edutopia.org, December 3, 2008.

Page 130 *"Beyond the Pill"*
Katz told me he hesitated to publicize High Tech High's success for
fear the schools would be flooded with parents of kids diagnosed
with ADD, yet as Parker revealed, that's a moot point. High Tech
High has already become a magnet for families struggling with children who have learning issues. "We're starting to worry about that,"
Parker told me, noting that the percentage of such kids has already
climbed from 6 to 14 percent in one of the schools.

Page 130 *In Virginia, a team of researchers*
The program, called Challenging Horizons, is led by psychology professor Steven Evans and paid for by big tobacco companies as part
of a statewide legal settlement.

Page 130 *Tools of the Mind*
The program is based on research conducted at the Metropolitan
State College of Denver.

Page 130 *an even simpler intervention—aerobic exercise*
See: John Ratey, *Spark: The Revolutionary New Science of Exercise
and the Brain* (Little, Brown and Company, 2008).

Page 131 *Universal Design for Learning*
A few months after I met Todd Rose, he was hired as a researcher
for CAST, the Center for Applied Special Technology, a nonprofit
organization that enthusiastically promotes the Universal Design for

Learning. CAST was founded in 1984 by the cognitive scientist David Rose, also quoted in this chapter.

At this writing, the Universal Design for Learning concept is gaining traction in U.S. schools. In a major milestone, the higher education bill passed in August of 2008 included an official definition of it, while five U.S. states have adopted various UDL policies, such as encouraging consideration of varying learning styles in textbook purchasing.

Page 132 *binge drinking*
Jim Staats, "Tamalpais School District Combats Teen Binge Drinking," *Marin Independent Journal,* March 4, 2009.

---

7. ADD-VOCACY

Page 134 *as if we're at a meeting of Alcoholics Anonymous*
The names of the speakers have been changed in the following quotes.

Page 135 *revenues of $4.2 million*
Similarly, the American Psychiatric Association received 28 percent of its revenues from drug firms from 2003 to 2008, according to an APA spokeswoman, although in the case of the APA, the trend is declining, due to increasing protests from members.

Page 141 *Blake Taylor*
See: Blake Taylor, *ADHD and Me: What I Learned from Lighting Fires at the Kitchen Table* (New Harbinger Publications, 2008).

Page 145 *significantly expanding the market for pharmaceutical stimulants*
CHADD moved to Landover, Maryland, in 1998, and two years later hired a longtime veteran disability-movement activist, E. Clarke Ross, the father of a son with ADD, to be its CEO. Ross had held positions including executive director of the American Managed Behavioral Healthcare Association and was well connected on Capitol Hill. His

efforts helped the group, in 2002, secure a $1 million grant from the Centers for Disease Control and Prevention to become, as CHADD's official history puts it, "a respected clearinghouse on science-based information."

Page 145 *three civil suits charging a conspiracy*
In 2000, plaintiffs' attorneys named CHADD as a co-conspirator, along with Novartis and the American Psychiatric Association, in a civil action consumer fraud case—variations of which were filed in at least three states. The lawyers charged the trio with joining to-gether to "invent and promote" the diagnosis of ADD so that the drug companies could profit from Ritalin sales. CHADD's activities, they said, had "led to a significant increase in the amount of Ritalin taken by school children and have directly resulted in enormous profits to the drug manufacturer."

Page 146 *Harvey Parker*
I interviewed Parker by phone in March of 2009. He has remained in Plantation, where three years after he helped launch CHADD's first chapter, he established a business called the "A.D.D. Warehouse," described on its Web site as "the world's largest collection of ADHD-related books, videos, training programs, games, professional texts and assessment products."

Page 146 *while drug-manufacturer support has increased*
Might CHADD be caught in a negative spiral, in which its damaged reputation has contributed to its declining membership, making it even more dependent on the drug firms, and further damaging its reputation? Might it finally reach the point that membership num-bers would be too low to continue with past limits on drug company support? CHADD CEO Ross declined my attempts to interview him on this subject, but spokesman Bryan Goodman said, "We deal with difficult issues as they arise, and the scenario you have presented is still strictly hypothetical," adding, "CHADD looks forward to a fu-ture of diversified funding."

Page 146 *dues-paying members had fallen to just twelve thousand*

There's a lot of confusion about CHADD's membership numbers. Harvey Parker told me the group had 40,000 members at its peak, which Goodman contradicted, saying organization records showed peak membership was 30,879 in 1997. And even that number may have been too high, Goodman told me, since the figure was read-justed to 24,013 in 1999 after the group automated its database. The membership number was readjusted yet again in 2002, when more technological changes were made, leading to a revised count of 19,766. Yet even with all those technological upgrades, the membership numbers continue to be a matter of dispute, at least among CHADD leaders. In the same month that Goodman told me CHADD had 12,000 members, the organization Web site gave a count of 20,000. At the Anaheim convention one month earlier, Anne Teeter Ellison told a workshop that there were 18,000 members.

Page 147 *9 million American adults*

This estimate was included in a McNeil Pediatrics press release, in September 2008, entitled "National Survey Reveals Impact of ADHD in Adults." I found it at http://www.mcneilpediatrics.net/mcneilpediatrics/assets/AdultADHDSurveyPressRelease_Final Sample.pdf.

Page 147 *trusted "most of the time"*

The survey was conducted by the Kaiser Family Foundation. See: "Drug Companies Temper Ads, Fear More FDA Rules," Associated Press, March 14, 2006. For a thorough investigation of modern phar-maceutical industry tactics, also see Melody Petersen's *Our Daily Meds: How the Pharmaceutical Companies Transformed Themselves into Slick Marketing Machines and Hooked the Nation on Prescription Drugs* (Farrar, Straus and Giroux, 2008). Petersen and other critics of the industry point out that Americans are already the world's most avid drug consumers, in part due to unrestrained lobbying by the drug firms. The industry, as Petersen reports, has spent more on lobbying the federal government in recent years than any other business, and by 2004, the companies employed so many lobbyists that there were more than two for each member of Congress.

Page 147 *"ADHD Moms"*
Initially, the Facebook page was hosted by middle school principal Debra Phelps, a familiar face to many as the mother of Olympic swimmer Michael Phelps. Debra Phelps vanished from the page in January 2009, however—the same month that photos were published of Michael with a bong. Both Phelps and a spokeswoman for McNeil say the two events were unrelated.

Page 148 *"drug holidays" are recommended by leading attention deficit experts*
See, for example: "3-Year Followup of the NIMH MTA Study," *Journal of the American Academy of Child & Adolescent Psychiatry* 46, no. 8 (August 2007): 989–1002. Interestingly enough, when I interviewed Debra Phelps, she said she personally opposed the common practice, at her school, of parents keeping children on meds without breaks.

Page 148 *tarnished by association*
The grass-roots group has had a few particularly embarrassing moments. One of these came in 1994, when it petitioned the U.S. Drug Enforcement Administration to relax restrictions on methylphenidate, the active ingredient in Ritalin. CHADD's position was understandable, in light of the difficulty its members must go through to get medication. The DEA classifies Ritalin as a "Schedule II" drug, along with opium and cocaine, due to the perceived risk of abuse. This means consumers have to get a new, written prescription every month that they use the drug. If your doctor doesn't trust you, or merely needs the income, he can make you return to his office every thirty days, obviously a costly and time-consuming commitment.

The DEA rules also limited production of methylphenidate, and as Ritalin sales surged in the early 1990s, supplies began to run out. CHADD was joined by the American Academy of Neurology in urging a change of the rules, and four other prestigious groups, including the American Psychiatric Association, endorsed the move. The DEA rebuffed them all, however, while a subsequent report by the United Nations International Narcotics Control Board warned that "treatment of ADD with Ritalin is being actively promoted by an influential 'parent association' that has received significant financial contributions from the leading manufacturer of this preparation in the United States."

No official U.S. action followed this alert, but the following year, Thomas Hehir, then director of the U.S. Department of Education's Office of Special Education, was "sandbagged" during a discussion of CHADD, as he told me in an interview, in a public TV documentary titled "ADD: A Dubious Diagnosis?" Hehir admired and worked closely with CHADD, which is why his department had recently commissioned the group to produce an ADD video for educators. But he also said he hadn't known anything about the group's drug-company funding until he was asked about it on camera. "It was quite a surprise," he said, fourteen years after the fact, in a telephone interview from his subsequent position, on the faculty at the Harvard Graduate School of Education. "We did not know that connection at that time and I felt frankly quite uncomfortable about it. The implication was we were pushing drugs on kids and families."

Hehir subsequently suspended dissemination of the video, which as he remembered included what he characterized as a responsible discussion of Ritalin as a treatment. "It wasn't the content of the video but the conflict of interest that was the problem for us," he said.

Page 148 *neurofeedback—a particularly controversial approach* CHADD in the past has ignored or sometimes opposed such alternative treatments. As recently as February 2008, an organization spokeswoman, Karen Sampson, told me the consensus of the group's expert advisors was that neurofeedback didn't work.

Page 149 *Some have had their trips paid for by pharmaceutical firms*

Willem de Jong, a psychologist and author from the Netherlands, told me his trip to the CHADD convention was paid for by Eli Lilly, which makes the ADD drug Strattera. In 2003, Eli Lilly, working with top U.S. ADD researcher Dr. Russell Barkley, also underwrote a new "Global Network" association of experts to raise awareness about the disorder outside the United States.

---

8. WIRED

Page 153 *increasingly widespread, high-tech therapy called neurofeedback*

Until the late 1960s, neurofeedback was mostly a subculture phenomenon, in which hippy therapists using big-box computers sought to help patients experience bliss by generating more of the relatively slow, "alpha" brain waves. Then, by means of a mix of smarts and luck, M. Barry Sterman, a research scientist at the University of California at Los Angeles, made a startling discovery. As Jim Robbins engagingly recounts in his book, *A Symphony in the Brain* (Grove Press, 2008), Sterman showed that neurofeedback training could protect cats—and, subsequently, humans—from seizures.

Sterman had been monitoring thirty lab cats to try to understand how the brain inhibits behavior. With electrodes attached to their scalps, the cats were trained to press a lever after waiting for a tone. Each time they performed correctly, they'd be rewarded with ladles of milk spiked with chicken broth. As they focused on their task, anticipating their reward, the cats became absolutely still, as if watching a mouse hole. Sterman's equipment recorded a brain-wave frequency that hadn't previously been described. At twelve to fifteen cycles per second, it was just faster than alpha, but barely at the next level, known as beta. He christened it sensory motor rhythm, or SMR.

Sterman trained his cats to generate SMR for up to four hours at a time. But then his funding dried up, most likely a casualty of federal grant-makers' general disdain for the fringy field. He had to move on, which is how he got that lucky break. His next project was to help NASA ascertain how exposure to the chemical hydrazine, in rocket fuel, might be affecting astronauts' brains. Sterman assembled another group of lab cats and injected them with the toxic substance. Most of the cats had seizures within two hours, and several of them died. But three survived, seizure-free. As Sterman soon realized, these hardy animals were the same cats he'd earlier trained in SMR. Somehow, the neurofeedback had strengthened their brains.

Sterman and colleagues eventually progressed to treating humans with epilepsy in a similar manner, and his reported success fanned interest in applying neurofeedback to other ailments. Eventually, Sterman trained several other clinicians, among them Cynthia Kerson and the University of Tennessee psychologist Joel Lubar, who in 1976 pioneered the use of neurofeedback for kids with ADD. Over the next couple of decades, Sterman's disciples joined other practitioner/researchers in producing more than one hundred scientific studies claiming positive results from the treatment, and by the first years of the New Millennium, the field was poised to explode.

Page 155 *"so amazing that nobody believes them"*
This quote appeared in Katy Butler's "Alice in Neuroland," in *Psychotherapy Networker,* September/October 2005. See also Hirshberg's review of neurofeedback studies: "EEG Biofeedback for ADHD: The State of the Evidence-Base," presented at the Annual Convention of the American Psychiatric Association, Toronto, Canada, in 2006. In recent years, dramatic testimonials about neurofeedback have indeed become abundant. See, for instance: *Ode Magazine*'s March 2009

story, "Improve Mental Health with Neurofeedback," by Baline Greteman, which includes a description of how John Gruzelier, a professor of psychology at the University of London's Goldsmiths College, has trained eye surgeons with the same technique used for kids with attention issues. Greteman reports that Gruzelier has enhanced the doctors' surgical performance by 20 percent, making them "slightly longer and more methodical in their preparatory time, then faster and more accurate on task."

Page 156 *"Based on previous reports, we're expecting attention to improve"*

Arnold told me one of the studies that most impressed him was by Roger deBeus, a researcher and private clinician as director of Advanced Psychological Services, in Hampton, Virginia. (See: R. deBeus, J. D. Ball et al., "Progress in Efficacy Studies of EEG Biofeedback for ADHD," a presentation at the Annual Meeting of the American Psychiatric Association, Toronto, Canada, May 2006.) For a critical review of recent research, see also "AD/HD and Neurofeedback: A Review of Eight Studies," from CHADD's National Resource Center, online at http://www.help4adhd.org/documents/Neurofeedback_8_Study_Review.pdf.

Page 156 *"The theory is that it will have a permanent effect"*

Arnold's study is intended to be the first neurofeedback research project to meet the "gold standard" of rigorous psychological research. Subjects are being randomly assigned to two groups, only one of which will be treated with genuine neurofeedback. Neither the subjects nor the researchers will know the difference until results are analyzed. The researchers are using software produced by SmartBrain Technologies in San Diego, California, involving a video game in which children make a car race ahead by generating desired brain-wave frequencies. For subjects in the "control" group, the effects will be random, meaning the car will race or stop independently of the quality of their brain waves. SmartBrain cofounder Lindsay Greco told me the technology was developed by NASA to train pilots in the late

1990s. NASA sold the license to her company in 2002. The equipment being used by federal researchers resembles the $595 units SmartBrain has been selling directly to consumers since 2005. It includes a visor with prearranged electrodes hooked into an iPod-like device that lets you choose between "improved concentration," "peak performance" for athletes, and a program to calm anxiety.

Page 157 *gamma waves*
Marc Kaufman, "Meditation Gives Brain a Charge, Study Finds," *Washington Post,* January 3, 2005.

Page 158 *270 U.S. deaths a day*
Melody Petersen, *Our Daily Meds* (Farrar, Straus and Giroux, 2008).

Page 159 *thirty times the amount of methylphenidate prescribed barely a decade ago*
In an interview in 2008, Pelham told me that he estimated that a typical ADD child who takes one of the newer, long-acting formulas and is medicated daily for a decade will consume nearly 150,000 mg of methylphenidate—fifteen to thirty times more than doses still common in the early 1990s. To be sure, very few children take the drugs for that long.

Page 159 *no more than eighteen months*
This estimate is from Peter Levine, MD, an ADD researcher in Kaiser Permanente's Department of Pediatrics in Walnut Creek, California.

Page 166 *it's not a universally accepted practice*
Lindsay Greco, the SmartBrain Technologies cofounder, says the decision about whether to send patients home with programmable technology is "one of the biggest ethical issues" in the field, since the programs can be changed inadvertently in ways that "aren't in your physiological interest." Over time, such changes can worsen an ADD disorder and/or increase anxiety, Greco told me.

Page 166 *tics, depression, "mental fogginess," seizures, panic attacks, incontinence*

Corydon Hammond and Lynda Kirk, "First, Do No Harm: Adverse Effects and the Need for Practice Standards in Neurofeedback," *Journal of Neurotherapy* 12, no. 1 (2008).

---

9. MEDITATION

Page 173 *may improve focus and curb impulsivity*

See, for example: Yi-Yuan Tang, Michael I. Posner et al., "Short-term Meditation Training Improves Attention and Self-regulation," *Proceedings of the National Academy of Sciences* 104, no. 43 (October 23, 2007). This study found that after just five days of training in a twenty-minute Chinese meditation technique, a randomly assigned team of eighty students scored better on tests of attention and mood and produced lower levels of the stress hormone cortisol while doing mental arithmetic, as compared to a group that was merely trained in muscle relaxation.

Additionally, University of California at Los Angeles researchers led by the attention deficit disorder expert Susan Smalley have reported that mindfulness training is a "feasible intervention" for some adults and adolescents with ADD and may help ameliorate difficulties in thinking and behavior. See: Lidia Zylowska et al., "Mindfulness Meditation Training in Adults and Adolescents with ADHD: A Feasibility Study," *Journal of Attention Disorders* 11, no. 6 (May 2008): 737–746.

Page 173 *entire families can benefit*

This brings up a point that has become increasingly clear to me as I've researched this book, which is that strategies aimed only at "fixing" a troubled child are rarely effective—particularly if that child's parents are coping with mental issues of their own. "In Western society, we're used to intervening with the child, be it with psychopharmaceuticals or behavioral training," the Buddhist psychologist

Nirbhay Singh told me. "But intervening in the transaction between the mother and child can be more helpful." Singh has gathered evidence of this with studies in which both children and mothers receive brief training in "mindfulness," the deliberate monitoring of attention, which has led, he says, to much more compliance by the children than when only the children are treated.

Page 175 *more than 10 million Americans*
Joel Stein, "Just Say Om," *Time,* August 4, 2003.

Page 175 *coaching students to count their breaths*
See, for example: www.innerkids.org.

One more sign of the times: at this writing, yoga has become a nearly $6 billion annual industry, according to Cassell Bryan, "Yoga Bears: It's No Stretch to Say Traders Are Taking Deep Breaths," *Wall Street Journal,* July 24, 2008.

Page 176 *those focus muscles*
A particularly intriguing study, published in 2005, found that long-time meditators actually have physically different brains—with relatively thicker parts of the cerebral cortex, involved in attention and sensory processing. (A caveat: it's not clear whether that apparently superior setup is the reason for or result of their disciplined practice.) See: S. W. Lazar et al., "Meditation Experience Is Associated with Increased Cortical Thickness," *Neuroreport,* no. 17 (November 28, 2005): 1893–1897.

Meanwhile, pathbreaking work by University of Toronto psychologist Zindel Segal has shown that a regular practice of "mindfulness" may prevent episodes of depression in patients with histories of recurrent mood disorder. Other research suggests the practice can help sharpen attention and even speed the healing of wounds and psoriasis. At this writing, Cliff Saron's Shamatha Project has illustrated measurable improvements for the obviously extra-motivated class of people willing to sit through three months of rigorous meditation

training. These include not only a greater capacity for sustained attention, but big reductions in depression, anxiety, sleep difficulties, and
hostility, Saron says. Saron's researchers at this writing are also track-
ing potential impacts on the levels of a vitally important enzyme
known as telomerase, which helps repair telomeres—the protective
caps on the ends of chromosomes—as they fray with age. The Nobel
Prize–winning cell biologist Elizabeth Blackburn, a biochemistry professor at the University of California at San Francisco, has collaborated in groundbreaking recent research involving mothers of seriously
ill children, which has shown that chronic stress appears to reduce
both the levels of telomerase and the length of telomeres. Blackburn
has been cooperating with Saron's team in looking at changes in
telomerase levels for participants in the Shamatha retreat. If benefits
are found, it will provide the most compelling evidence yet that we
can use our minds to change our physical makeup, right down to the
molecular level.

Page 176 *"blissing out under a bongo tree"*
I interviewed the whimsical Ricard for a story on meditation in the
September/October 2006 issue of *Psychology Today* titled "Mastering
Your Own Mind."

Page 181 *"suffering a knee-slapper"*
Perry Garfinkel, "Joke's Not Funny? Blame It on Buddha," *New York
Times,* September 2, 2003.

Page 182 *colored disk on his forehead*
Steve Heilig, "Wes 'Scoop' Nisker: Keeping the Faith in More Ways
Than One," *San Francisco Chronicle,* April 13, 2003.

Page 183 *"We are disturbed"*
Epictetus is quoted in Gordon Peerman, *Blessed Relief: What Chris-
tians Can Learn from Buddhists About Suffering* (SkyLight Paths
Publishing, 2008).

Page 186 *talking about summoning compassion*

Douglas and other meditation teachers remind us that the practice of nurturing compassion for others begins with being able to be compassionate to yourself. In recent years, psychologists have turned their attention to this skill of "self-compassion." In 2007, for instance, Duke University scientists reported findings suggesting that a broad definition of self-compassion, including a capacity to simply let go of painful thoughts, was more helpful than self-esteem in making people resilient.

Buddhists teach that once you've mastered compassion for yourself, you can progress to include strangers and eventually even people you've thought of as enemies. Ideally, so the theory goes, at some point something shifts so that you no longer need to be meditating to do this. As Matthieu Ricard describes it, "It's like riding a horse. In the beginning you have to be very careful not to fall off, but pretty soon you even forget you're on a horse."

Page 189 *who painted the sky*

Researchers who study meditation and neurofeedback have described this sensation as the "clean windshield" effect.

---

10. THE WHITE CONTENDER

Page 195 *"Buddhism is an evolutionary sport"*

From Richard Schreinin, "Scholar Robert Thurman Trades His Western Ego for a Buddhist Self," Knight-Ridder Newspapers, March 20, 1996.

Page 196 *with the timely theme of nurturing compassion in children*

The Seeds of Compassion conference took place under the auspices of the Kirlin Foundation, somewhat ironically established by the Bellevue, Washington, beeper-and-cell-phone mogul and philanthropist Dan Kranzler. The conference also drew support from several of the state's leading political and religious leaders.

Page 199 *he takes lithium*
Lisa Katayama, "Interview with Dalai Lama's Younger Brother," *Asian Window,* September 1, 2008.

Page 199 *channeling the Tibetan sage*
In my conversation with Saron about whether the Dalai Lama would approve of medications for mental illness, he mentioned that he once heard a psychiatrist ask his opinion of the "unnatural" intervention of gene therapy, to which Tenzin Gyatso replied: "You think the Buddhist path of mind training is natural?"

Page 199 *"all the love and care in the world is unlikely to fix a leaky synapse"*
Writing about meditation and antidepressants in "Awakening with Prozac," an article in the fall 1993 edition of *Tricycle,* the New York psychiatrist and practicing Buddhist Mark Epstein observed that "to suffer from psychiatric illness willfully, when treatment is mercifully available, is but a contemporary ascetic practice." It may also interfere with emotional and spiritual growth, as Epstein suggested, noting that when depressed people try to meditate, "instead of letting it take them forward, they're using their meditation as an attempt to self-medicate. The bulk of their energy may go into obsessive ruminations or attempts to process emotional pain that feels stuck. They are facing a gradient that is too steep."

Page 199 *"no need to worry"*
This quote can be found on the Dalai Lama's Web site, at www .dalailama.com/page.54.htm. Not only is there no benefit in worrying, researchers point out that there's much potential harm. Worry, as many recent studies have confirmed, corrodes the brain, dousing it with stress hormones that diminish capacity for memory and focus.

However unfair this may seem for those of us who feel it's our duty to shoulder the weight of the world, people who manage to avoid self-doubt and worry are often not only healthier but happier and more successful. See, for example: the interesting paper "Self-Deception and Its Relationship to Success in Competition," by Joanna E. Starek and Caroline F. Keating, in *Basic and Applied Social Psychology* 12, no. 2 (1991): 145–155. "Our motivation to negotiate daily life depends on some degree of misplaced optimism about what we are capable of accomplishing," the authors note.

Page 205 *a new era of understanding*
Mothers and neuroscientists may lead the way here. We mothers, after all, have the most hardwired motivation of all to see our children in the most hopeful light. For some of us, at least, that means we'll end up following the compassionate principle so eloquently expressed by child psychologist Ross Greene (author of *The Explosive Child*, Harper Paperbacks, 2005), that *all* "challenging behavior" stems from lagging skills and unsolved problems. Neuroscientists, meanwhile, are steadily helping us appreciate the biological basis of so much behavior we've traditionally chalked up to plain badness. One striking and extreme example is the case of recent research into the nature of psychopaths. See, for instance: John Seabrook, "Suffering Souls," *New Yorker,* November 10, 2008. Seabrook profiles the neuroscientist Kent Kiehl, who complains that there is much more research funding available to study schizophrenics, since, unlike psychopaths, they're seen as victims, even as brain scans of psychopaths suggest their "evil" natures stem from a breakdown in communication between the frontal lobes and deeper parts of the brain, affecting attention and inhibition—the same functions that are impaired, albeit to a lesser degree, in attention deficit disorder. As with clinical distraction, psychopathic behavior is now presumed to start with genes, yet isn't predestined—as with ADD, there's evidence it can be aggravated in neglectful families.

EPILOGUE: WHAT ELSE WORKED

Page 218 *fish oil*

See, for example: "Omega-3 Fatty Acids in ADHD and Related Neurodevelopmental Disorders," *International Review of Psychiatry* 18, no. 2 (April 2006): 155–172.

It's important to remember that the quality of supplements varies. Look for a brand that specifies that the oil is free of mercury and has a good ratio of the two major fatty acids: eicosapentaenoic acid (EPA) and docosahexaenoic acid (DHA). Scientists recommend three times the amount of EPA to DHA.

Page 219 *Experts recommend*

Dr. Edward Hallowell suggests this dose in his book *Delivered from Distraction* (Ballantine, 2005).

Page 219 *shakes that were taken off the market*

The shakes were made by Sunrider International. Salmonella can cause nausea, fever, headache, diarrhea, and vomiting in healthy adults, and can be fatal to infants and to elderly or debilitated people.

Page 219 *ginkgo biloba and/or ginseng*

Ian K. Smith, MD, "A Dangerous Mix," *Time*, October 9, 2000.

Page 219 *artificial colors and flavors, as well as benzoate preservative*

D. McCann et al., "Food Additives and Hyperactive Behaviour in 3-year-old and 8/9-year-old Children in the Community: A Randomised, Double-blinded, Placebo-controlled Trial," *Lancet* 370, no. 9598 (November 3, 2007): 1560–1567. In 2009, the state of Maryland was considering outlawing these chemicals in schools.

Page 219 *even low-level contact with the common insecticides known as organophosphates*

Joel T. Nigg, *What Causes ADHD: Understanding What Goes Wrong and Why* (Guilford Press, 2006).

Page 219 *exercise stands out*

See, for example: John Ratey, *Spark: The Revolutionary New Science of Exercise and the Brain* (Little, Brown and Company, 2008), and also Debra Viadero, "Exercise Seen as Priming Pump for Students' Academic Strides," *Education Week,* February 12, 2008.

Page 220 *"God's Recipe"*

FTC press release, "Multi-Level Marketing Company to Settle FTC Charges That It Made Unsubstantiated Claims That Its 'God's Recipe' Dietary Regimen Could Cure ADD/ADHD," December 8, 1998.

Page 220 *hair samples for analysis*

The method is extremely controversial, according to sources including the book *Healing the New Childhood Epidemics*, by Kenneth Bock, MD (Random House, 2008). Additionally, a report published in *JAMA,* the *Journal of the American Medical Association,* in 2001, revealed that on average, hair-analysis lab reports were unreliable. See: Steven J. Steindel, PhD, and Peter J. Howanitz, MD, "The Uncertainty of Hair Analysis for Trace Metals," *JAMA* 285 (2001): 83–85.

Page 220 *the "Dore Method"*

The method is named for Wynford Dore, a wealthy entrepreneur whose daughter reportedly struggled with dyslexia. Dore assembled a team of scientists who devised the exercise program with the primary goal of stimulating the cerebellum, a brain region known to be involved in coordination, working memory, attention, and impulse control. The cerebellum has also been identified as one of the brain structures tending to be underdeveloped in children diagnosed with ADD. In the year I spent reporting this book, however, Dore programs were closing down and going bankrupt, as subscriptions plummeted.

Page 221 *a "balance board"*

I owe thanks to Sue Smalley, who suggested this purchase.

Page 221 *researchers trained preschool children*
M. Rosario Rueda et al., "Training, Maturation, and Genetic Influences on the Development of Executive Attention," *Proceedings of the National Academy of Sciences* 102, no. 41 (October 11, 2005): 14931–14936.

Page 222 *Nirbhay Singh*
See: "Individuals with Mental Illness Can Control Their Aggressive Behavior Through Mindfulness Training," *Behavior Modification* 31, no. 3 (May 2007): 313–328.

Page 224 *deviancy-training workshop*
This is how Dr. Russell Barkley referred to the classes in the February 2008 lecture I attended.

SELECT BIBLIOGRAPHY

Barkley, Dr. Russell. *Taking Charge of ADHD: The Complete, Authoritative Guide for Parents.* Guilford Press, 2000.

Breggin, Dr. Peter. *Talking Back to Ritalin: What Doctors Aren't Telling You About Stimulants and ADHD.* Perseus Publishing, 2001.

Cohn, Art. *The Nine Lives of Michael Todd.* Pocket Books, 1959.

Demos, John. *Getting Started with Neurofeedback.* W.W. Norton & Co., 2005.

Greene, Ross. *The Explosive Child: Understanding and Helping Easily Frustrated, "Chronically Inflexible" Children.* Harper Paperbacks, 2005.

Hallowell, Dr. Edward, and Dr. John Ratey. *Driven to Distraction: Recognizing and Coping with Attention Deficit Disorder from Childhood Through Adulthood.* Touchstone, 1994.

Hartmann, Thom. *Beyond ADD: Hunting for Reasons in the Past and Present.* Underwood Books, 1996.

Hirstein, William. *Brain Fiction: Self-Deception and the Riddle of Confabulation.* MIT Press, 2005.

Honos-Webb, Lara. *The Gift of ADHD: How to Transform Your Child's Problems into Strengths.* New Harbinger Publications, 2005.

Jackson, Maggie. *Distracted: The Erosion of Attention and the Coming Dark Age.* Prometheus Books, 2008.

Jackson, Philip. *Life in Classrooms.* Teachers College Press, 1990.

Klingberg, Torkel. *The Overflowing Brain: Information Overload and the Limits of Working Memory.* Oxford University Press, 2009.

Lipton, Bruce. *The Biology of Belief: Unleashing the Power of Consciousness, Matter, and Miracles.* Mountain of Love, 2005.

Louv, Richard. *Last Child in the Woods: Saving Our Children from Nature-Deficit Disorder.* Atlantic Books, 2009.

Petersen, Melody. *Our Daily Meds: How the Pharmaceutical Companies Transformed Themselves into Slick Marketing Machines and Hooked the Nation on Prescription Drugs.* Farrar, Straus and Giroux, 2008.

Ratey, Dr. John. *Spark: The Revolutionary New Science of Exercise and the Brain.* Little, Brown and Company, 2008.

Robbins, Jim. *A Symphony in the Brain: The Evolution of the New Brain Wave Biofeedback.* Grove Press, 2008.

Taylor, Blake. *ADHD and Me: What I Learned from Lighting Fires at the Kitchen Table.* New Harbinger Publications, 2008.

Tyre, Peg. *The Trouble with Boys: A Surprising Report Card on Our Sons, Their Problems at School, and What Parents and Educators Must Do.* Crown, 2008.

Wallace, B. Alan. *The Attention Revolution: Unlocking the Power of the Focused Mind.* Wisdom Publications, 2006.

Whybrow, Dr. Peter. *American Mania: When More Is Not Enough.* W.W. Norton & Company, 2005.

On Methods and
In Gratitude

The majority of the events in this book took place between September 2007 and September 2008, beginning with my argument with Buzz on the highway and ending with his becoming a bar mitzvah. The main exceptions are the scenes in Chapter 2, detailing events leading up to our decision on medication, which Buzz began in the early summer of 2006, and in Chapter 7, describing my attendance with Buzz at the CHADD convention, in November 2008.

There are no invented scenes or dialogue, but I have changed some names and, in a few cases, some details. I gave my two children pseudonyms because although I hope they'll be proud of their stories as I've written them, it also seemed right to offer a buffer in terms of electronic database searchability. As indicated in the text and endnotes, I also changed the names of friends with children diagnosed with ADD, and of therapists who treated us who weren't public figures—i.e., all of them, except for Dr. Daniel Amen and Cynthia Kerson. In Chapter 3, due to copyright laws, I was obliged to change the gist of the questions on the neuropsychological tests "Rachel Brown" gave to Buzz, and, necessarily, also his answers.

TO BE FRANK, initially, I wasn't sure—*what else is new?*—that writing this book was such a great idea. I'd never published anything this personal about myself or my children, and I worried about the future consequences for Buzz. On the other hand, at the time I made my decision to move forward, back in September 2007, the level of conflict in our family was still extreme, despite how much Buzz's behavior had improved with medication. I also still felt huge reservations about relying on the meds without exploring alternative treatments, and didn't feel I sufficiently understood the trade-offs and risks involved. There was so much that I needed to learn, with so little time that I could afford to take from other work, and so much danger that I'd get distracted by other projects until the next crisis hit. Thus, I came to see the book project as an irresistible opportunity to fix my focus, with the grappling hooks of writing deadlines, on finding a way out.

I realize, even so, that not every reader will approve of my decision to write about my family in this way. I entertained my own anguished doubts—particularly concerning whether Buzz was old enough to give his informed consent to this project—right up until the night that we hashed out the terms of his cooperation.

At Buzz's insistence, we held our meeting at a Mill Valley steak house he'd spotted from the highway. Buzz donned his hand-me-down Ralph Lauren blazer, and I, in a rare concession, wore a dress and high heels. Once seated at our table, he coolly waved off a waitress's attempt to hand him a child's menu and crayons, and proceeded to order the $29.95 New York steak with the blue-cheese rosti, served rare. Before the food arrived, he got right to the point. He'd help me out, he said, but he wanted half of the proceeds from the book, including foreign sales. Pre-tax.

By dessert—ginger cake soaked in chocolate sauce—I'd shaken off my worries about whether I might be exploiting my vulnerable son, and, with great effort, talked him down to 10 percent, some of which could be spent on his private school tuition and future college education.

I drew up a contract, which we both signed, and which I taped to my office wall. It stipulated Buzz's deliverables: among other things, he'd have to make an effort to communicate with me, to participate in neurofeedback and meditation training, and attend a reasonable number of sessions with therapists. Part of the payment would be placed in a college savings account, and per explicit agreement, Buzz would forfeit the rest were he to be suspended from school and/or seriously injure his brother.

I'm proud to report that Buzz to date has fulfilled his part of this agreement, and to vow that he can count on me to fulfill mine.

AS FOR THE obvious question of how I could finish writing *any* book while coping with a high-maintenance family and my own clinical-grade distraction, here are my two main secrets: Being obsessed. And having extraordinarily insightful and generous relatives and friends.

I intend to spend a lot of time and energy thanking all of them in person, but for the record, they are:

My family: including my husband, Jack Epstein; parents Dr. Ellis and Bernice Ellison; and siblings Dr. David Ellison, Dr. James Ellison, and Dr. Jean Milofsky.

Dear friends: Claudia Belshaw, Nancy Boughey, Michelle Bullard, Joanna Caplan, Emily Goldfarb, Sharon Lape, Dr. John Ruark, Elizabeth Share, Diana Velasquez, and Jill Wolfson.

I also so appreciate the following publishing professionals who supported this book with talent and enthusiasm: Elizabeth Crane, Pamela Dorman, Barbara Jones, Michelle Tessler, Catherine Thorpe, Leslie Wells, and, with especially fervent gratitude, the eagle-eyed copyeditor, Rick Willett.

My continuing gratitude goes to the newspaper editors who didn't fire me when they had the chance: John Baker, Pat Dillon, and Bob Ryan.

Also, huge thanks to the psychologists, psychiatrists, neuroscientists, and other experts who patiently helped me to understand complicated subjects: Dr. Daniel Amen, Dr. Russell Barkley, Dr. Jim Dimon, Virginia Douglas, Dr. Glenn Elliott, Cynthia Kerson, Michael Posner, Cynthia Peterson, Ilina Singh, Nirbhay Singh, Susan Smalley, and B. Alan Wallace.

Finally, I want to give special recognition to the following people, whose extraordinary support helped make this book truly a labor of love. The list starts with my writers' group, N. 24th, wise, bighearted women who saw this book through from idea to manuscript: Allison Bartlett, Leslie Crawford, Frances Dinkelspiel, Sharon Epel, Susan Freinkel, Katherine Neilan, Lisa Okuhn, Julia Flynn Siler, and Jill Storey. It also includes my dear brother Dr. James Ellison, and the amazing Katy Butler, Stephen Hinshaw, Todd Rose, and Cliff Saron.

Index